DISEASES
IN HISTORY
Flu

Diseases in History
FLU

Kevin Cunningham

MORGAN REYNOLDS

PUBLISHING

Greensboro, North Carolina

Diseases in History

PLAGUE

FLU

MALARIA

HIV/AIDS

Library of Congress Cataloging-in-Publication Data

Cunningham, Kevin, 1966-
    Diseases in history. Flu / by Kevin Cunningham.
        p. cm.
    Includes bibliographical references and index.
    ISBN-13: 978-1-59935-105-6
    ISBN-10: 1-59935-105-6
    1. Influenza--History. I. Title. II. Title: Flu.
    RC150.1.C86 2009
    614.5'18--dc22

                                        2008051620

Printed in the United States of America
First Edition

Contents

Introduction

*I*n Atlanta, in a freezer behind a high-tech security array, the Centers for Disease Control guards one of history's deadliest killers: the mysterious disease that in 1918 and 1919 struck down its victims like nothing else in memory.

Healthy young adults became deathly ill in a matter of hours. A victim's ears and lips turned blue. Soon the skin turned the same color. As the disease advanced, the fingertips and feet turned black. Blood streamed from the nose and gums, and was coughed up in thick sputum that soaked a victim's pillows and bed sheets. The lungs were virtually turned into pulp by the virus and the immune system's attempt to kill it. Alternately sweating and shaking with chills, the victim died gasping for air, his desperate breaths sounding like crinkling paper.

Sometimes it killed in weeks, sometimes less than twenty-four hours.

Known as the Spanish flu, the epidemic blazed for eighteen months and killed between 40 and 100 million human beings. Then it vanished.

Focused on World War I and its stormy aftermath, and perhaps eager to forget the disease, people let the Spanish flu fade from memory.

In a way, that was typical. Influenza has always traveled through history with a low profile.

One reason is a lack of medical knowledge. Even in 1918, no human being had ever seen a virus. Human influenza wasn't isolated in the laboratory until years later, in 1933.

Another reason is influenza's symptoms. On the whole they are considered unremarkable: headaches, fever and chills, a runny nose, a heavy chest. Most of the time, we catch a flu virus, suffer for a few days, and get better. Often we're even not aware we had influenza because it shares its symptoms with so many minor ailments.

Influenza's names have been colorful, though. Medieval Italians called it the *influenza di freddo* (influence of the cold) when it arrived during winter weather and just the *influence* when they blamed it on an unfavorable alignment of certain stars and planets.

The British called it "knock-me-down fever" or, with English dry wit, "the new acquaintance." To the French it was "*la grippe*;" to the Germans the "*blitzkatarrh*;" to the Persians "the disease of the wind;" and to the Japanese "*kanbo*." Other names included "catarrh" and "the grip."

For years, Americans have used the word *flu* to describe an unpleasant but mild illness. Nausea or vomiting is "stomach flu." A bad cough or cold, perhaps with a slight fever, is just "the flu."

However, it's inaccurate to use *flu* or *influenza* as a catchall term for minor ailments. Influenza is not diarrhea. It is not a cold that spins out of control.

The term *influenza* describes a disease caused by a puffball-shaped virus of the *Orthomyxoviridae* family. When our discussion here refers to influenza or flu, we specifically mean that virus or disease. Unless noted, it also refers to Type A influenza, the fast-mutating and most dangerous form.

Humanity has conquered or curbed many diseases in the last century. Influenza remains undefeated. It is an astonishingly complex adversary—wildly contagious, ever-changing and secretive, at times only aggravating, at other times a ferocious killer. In fact, we are just now beginning to understand how the virus works.

One of influenza's most amazing traits is its ability to kill without setting off alarms.

In the United States, a country with excellent medical care and the world's mightiest economy, influenza remains a serious public health problem. Of the top ten causes of death, it is the only infectious disease on the list. Most Americans are unaware that influenza kills from 36,000 to 50,000 people in the United States every year. The exact number is elusive. Flu is so tricky that the Center for Disease Control (CDC), the hub of the U.S. public health system, cannot get an accurate count.

Worldwide, an estimated 100 million people catch influenza in an average year, with an estimated 1 million dying. But these figures are little more than educated guesses. The lack of statistics from major countries like China and India make the real count uncertain. Poorer nations lack the means to gather data. Furthermore, several diseases common in tropical nations, like malaria, cause headaches, fevers, and other flu-like symptoms, confusing anyone trying to count.

Today we face a new and dangerous form of the disease. In scientific shorthand these influenza viruses are called H5N1. People know it better as avian influenza, or the bird flu. Since its initial appearance in 1997, H5N1 has spread throughout Asia, to northern and western Africa, and to Europe. On occasion, it infects human beings. As of January 2009, more than two hundred fifty people had died. And no one believes H5N1 will go away anytime soon.

In fact, scientists fear avian influenza will mutate into a form capable of spreading from person to person. That's how the Spanish flu spread in 1918. The result in the twenty-first century might be just as devastating.

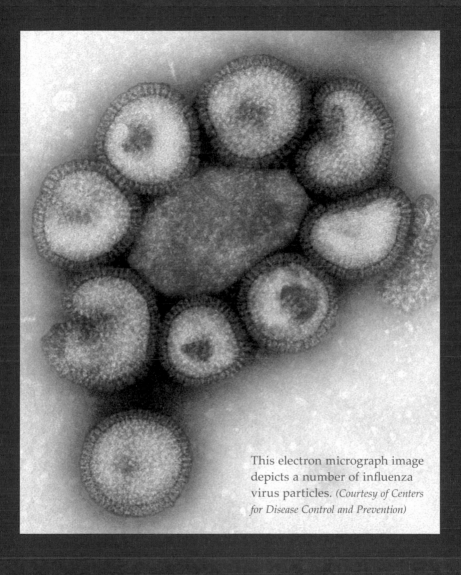

This electron micrograph image depicts a number of influenza virus particles. *(Courtesy of Centers for Disease Control and Prevention)*

one
Ever-Changing Virus

Diseases of animals often cross over to *Homo sapiens*. More than eight hundred human diseases, including many of the major epidemic illnesses, originated in animals. Bubonic plague, the terror of the Middle Ages and the Renaissance, came from rodents. Measles, it is thought, crossed over from dogs. Bizarre new diseases like Ebola, the hemorrhaging fever of Central Africa, most likely come from an unknown animal (or animals).

The influenza virus evolved in waterfowl, a group of bird species that includes geese, swans, terns, and gulls. In all likelihood, however, influenza has its origin in ducks. Of the birds the virus infects, it seems to have adapted best to the duck's body, especially to the intestines and the respiratory tract.

Under most circumstances, influenza doesn't harm ducks or other birds. Today, migrating waterfowl carry all the

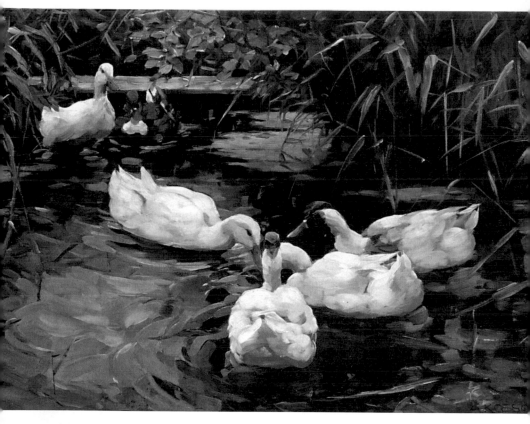

An 1890 painting of ducks by Alexander Koester. Evidence suggests that the influenza virus first evolved in waterfowl, specifically ducks.

known subtypes of influenza virus, suggesting that it's been inside those species a long time, probably for millions of years.

It's impossible to know when influenza leapt from birds into human history. The likeliest explanation is that the human-flu relationship began in the early days of agriculture. Close contact between farmers and their livestock inaugurated the era of animal diseases finding a way into human beings.

In many places, a farmer not only kept animals, he lived with them. Livestock was valuable property. The wise owner brought his animals inside during storms or shared his farmhouse with them during the winter. Human beings soon began to catch diseases from pigs and the whole range of domesticated animals: sheep, cattle, goats, ducks, chickens, geese, camels, and horses. Viruses and bacteria also jumped from the dogs and cats people took as companions, and from the rodents that ate their grain.

Experts theorize that influenza first entered human society in China. Chinese farmers have kept domesticated ducks

A chicken vendor resting on top of chicken cages at a market in Shanghai, China. *(Courtesy of AP Images)*

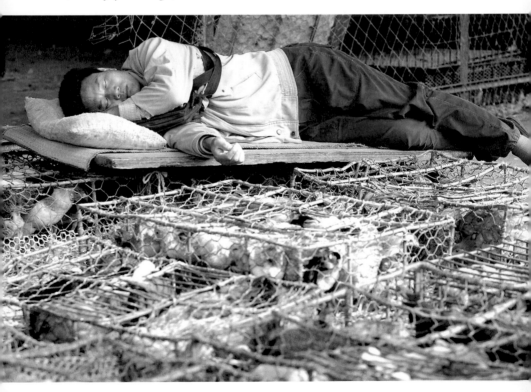

for centuries. Ducks found an agreeably watery home on rice paddies. During growing season, the ducks left the rice plants alone. Afterward, they pecked fallen grains out of the mud for food. All the while, the ducks excreted influenza virus in their feces into the water.

Possibly the disease found its way into pigs, a common livestock animal in China, and one prone to rooting around in the mud where ducks left their waste. An avian form of influenza cannot always link to human cells (though some may be better at it than others). But bird flu has an easier time infecting pigs. It's possible influenza slowly adapted to swine. It then had a better chance of infecting human farmers, because pigs and human beings share about 70 percent of their DNA.

That's one theory, anyway. We have no way of knowing if it happened that way. In fact, it's not certain influenza infected pigs at all before 1918. New flu viruses, however, do evolve by that method today. Ducks and pigs live side-by-side in China, just as they have for centuries. This provides excellent conditions for various kinds of flu to trade genetic material and create hybrid viruses.

In fact, these agricultural practices are a major reason the scientific community believes new influenza strains originate in southern China. Of the known pandemic-causing flu viruses, all appeared first in that region (with the exception of the Spanish flu in 1918). The Chinese, not appreciating the association with a deadly disease, resist the idea. But influenza experts spend a lot of time and effort watching the country to see what viruses emerge.

New viruses seldom cause problems, in us or in animals. As a researcher at the National Institute of Health explains,

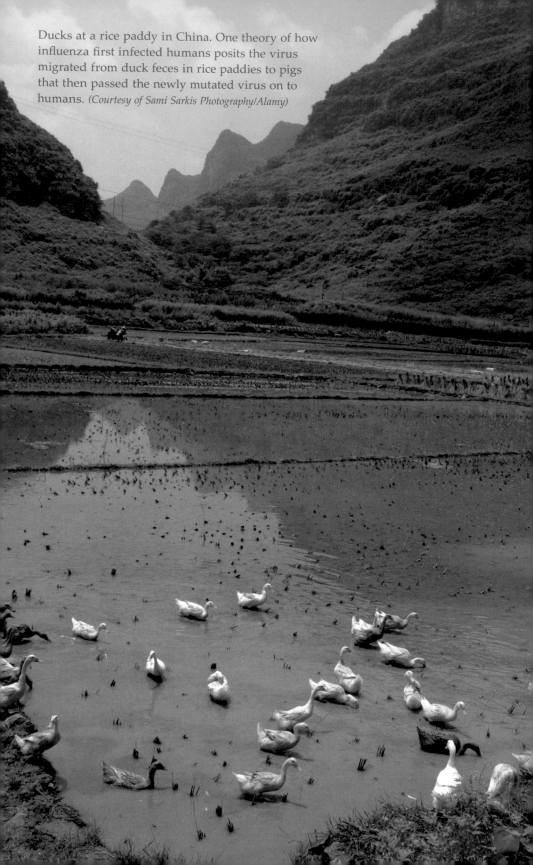

Ducks at a rice paddy in China. One theory of how influenza first infected humans posits the virus migrated from duck feces in rice paddies to pigs that then passed the newly mutated virus on to humans. *(Courtesy of Sami Sarkis Photography/Alamy)*

"the vast majority of [hybrids] between avian and human (or mammalian) influenza viruses contain a gene . . . or [group of genes] that prevents the virus replicating efficiently in primates."

If that weren't the case, we'd have to deal with one influenza pandemic after another.

Influenza belongs to the *Orthomyxoviridae* family. There are three types.

Type C can, but seldom does, cause humans to become seriously ill.

Type B influenza tends to be more aggravating than dangerous—though it can kill in certain cases. It circulates in predictable low-key viruses.

Type A influenza is unpredictable. It often is mild, but at times is deadly and the cause of flu pandemics. Type A encompasses a huge range of viruses. In addition to the "bird flu" currently spreading around the world, Type A includes swine flu and human viruses. These viruses change their genetic structure from generation to generation—or mutate— at a fast rate. Partly because of that, influenza continuously baffles the human immune system; it's the reason a flu vaccine that works one year becomes worthless the next.

Scientists break down influenza's evolution into two categories.

Antigenic drift describes the constant changes in a flu virus's genetic structure through mutation. Sometimes the mutation is slow; at other times it is dramatic and fast. An influenza virus drifts because it cannot copy itself accurately.

The genes of some viruses sit on a double-stranded molecule in the shape of a spiral staircase—the double helix of deoxyribonucleic acid, or DNA. But influenza's genes are coded on ribonucleic acid, or RNA, a simpler, single-stranded molecule.

RNA doesn't have the mechanism that DNA uses to "edit" itself during the replication process. As a result, each copy of an influenza virus contains errors. A misplaced amino acid here. A dropped fragment there. The errors add up as the virus, and its flawed descendants continue to reproduce. Eventually, the genes change, or drift, into a new form.

Since the genetic blueprint determines every aspect of influenza's existence, the virus changes too, both in structure and behavior. Over longer periods, antigenic drift transforms a virus altogether. The distant descendants of the terrible Spanish flu circulate today, but are so changed that they're not considered a threat.

Influenza also changes through antigenic shift, a rarer and more radical change.

If two different influenza viruses infect the same animal—for instance, a pig—genetic material from one can mix part of its genetic material with that of the other. The result is a new flu virus. Scientists call the process reassortment (or genetic reassortment).

Imagine someone has thrown playing cards into a hat. Ten red-suited cards represent the ten genes of the first influenza virus. Ten black-suited cards represent the genes of a second. Drawing ten at random gives you a hand made up of cards— genes—from each. In other words, a whole new virus made up of a mixture of red genes and black genes.

For a long time, the most dangerous reassortments were thought to take place inside a pig. Because swine catch both human and avian influenza, it seemed most likely that a pig, of all animals, would catch a human virus and a bird virus at the same time. The two would exchange genetic material and a new, reassorted virus then jumped from the pig and infected human beings.

Scientists have learned that a human being can also host a genetic reassortment. It would work the same way. A person sick with (human) flu somehow catches an avian virus and the two combine, with the result an exotic bird flu able to spread among humans. Since human beings have no immunity to avian influenza, such a virus would represent a tremendous threat to life.

A second kind of antigenic shift occurs when an avian virus mutates into a form that allows it to jump straight from birds to people without a reassortment being involved. When this occurs, the virus evolves within the victim's body into a form that can more efficiently link up with human cells. The new form then gets passed to other people, and they pass it to others. Throughout the process, the virus continues to mutate toward a form that spreads person-to-person.

The virus capable of this genetic sorcery looks like a cotton ball. Influenza is, as viruses go, small. Ten thousand or so virions strung together would equal one millimeter.

A forest of proteins covers the surface of the membrane surrounding the virus's ten genes. Two of the proteins predominate.

Hemagglutinin, abbreviated to HA or H, resembles a shaft or spike. Its partner, *neuraminidase* (NA or N), looks like a mushroom or sledgehammer.

At present, we know of sixteen distinct types of HA proteins and nine distinct types of NA proteins. Scientists identify each with a simple numeric system—H1 through H16,

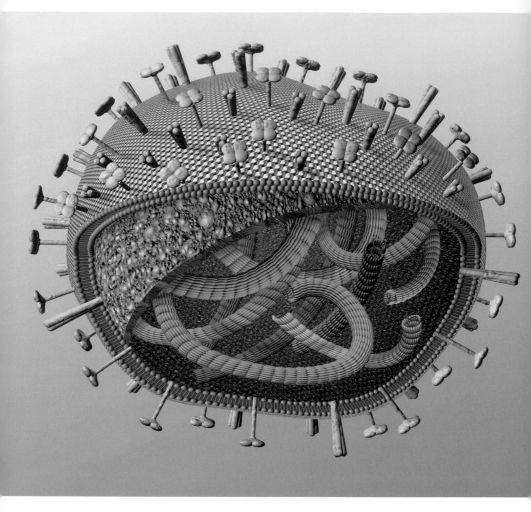

A three-dimensional rendering of the influenza virus. Strands of RNA inhabit the interior of the virus, while the outside is covered with hemagglutinin proteins (shaped like spikes) and neuraminidase proteins (shaped like mushrooms). *(Courtesy of Phototake Inc./Alamy)*

and N1 through N9. A flu virus carries one specific kind of HA and one kind of NA. A kind of influenza with the H5 hemagglutinin protein and the N1 neuraminidase protein would be labeled H5N1.

Such abbreviations are used for each influenza A subtype, the families of viruses that make up the influenza universe.

There are thousands of viruses (called strains) within a sub-type. While part of the same family, the viruses within a single subtype may vary a great deal.

For example, the bird flu in the news belongs to the H5N1 subtype. One of the H5N1 viruses, the Z+ strain, is among the most lethal forms of influenza ever studied. Yet other H5N1s circulate in wild birds without causing serious illness, or any illness at all.

An influenza virus first invades the epithelial cells lining the nose and throat. The protective cell wall, one of our outer defenses against disease, dies and sloughs off. Even as this is happening a victim feels fine. Symptoms show up in one to three days, though it may take as long as six. Usually a person becomes contagious in about twenty-four hours and remains so for three to four days.

A flu victim deals with varying levels of misery. A mild case may mean a sore throat and runny nose, a headache or pains in the joints. It might keep a person off work or out of school for a day or two. Many people, however, tough it out—and therefore cough, sneeze, and breathe virus onto co-workers, fellow students, people on the bus, or anyone else they come into contact with.

Severe influenza causes those symptoms but may also trigger a high fever, cause patients to cough up bloody liquid, or develop into fatal pneumonia. The Spanish influenza and some of today's H5N1 bird flu viruses produce even more dangerous symptoms.

Not every infected person shows symptoms, however. A substantial number show none. Doctors refer to these people as asymptomatic. Asymptomatic victims carry the virus and are still contagious. During the Spanish influenza pandemic, about 28 percent of Americans got sick, to one degree or another. But at least a third, and probably more, caught the virus and didn't know it.

In the Northern Hemisphere, flu season arrives with late autumn's cold and damp weather. Tens of millions catch the disease every year. Most recover. That said, even a mild flu virus poses risks to certain groups. Older people can and do die of influenza that a teenager will shake off. That's the reason why vaccination campaigns aim at the elderly. Babies and toddlers are also vulnerable, as are those with weak immune systems, such as people with AIDS.

In much of the world, flu is endemic, that is, constantly present in a population. On occasion, a virus flares up to cause an epidemic—an above-average number of cases in an area or country. Often this happens during influenza season. Since few people die, these epidemics rarely make it to the television news.

But three to five times per century, a Type A virus undergoes an extreme change. These extraordinary and dangerous viruses cause pandemics. Pandemics, unlike epidemics, are worldwide outbreaks of a disease. Pandemic influenza kills not thousands or hundreds of thousands but millions. Rather than flaring briefly, a pandemic can last months or even years.

What's in a Name?

At first glance, the name of a specific flu virus can appear intimidating—an alphabet soup of words, letters, and numbers, with the occasional slash thrown in to add to the confusion. The naming system used by scientists, however, conveys a great deal of information in a small amount of space.

The name of an influenza virus takes into account:

* Type of influenza. (A or B—Type C viruses are not given names)
* Animal host, if other than human. (For instance, swine or avian.)
* The place where it was discovered.
* A classification number.
* The year of discovery.
* The number of the virus's HA protein (H) and NA protein (N).

For example, A/swine/Maryland/16/07 [H7N2] is a Type A swine influenza virus discovered in Maryland, classified number sixteen, found in 2007; and belonging to the subtype H7N2, a family of viruses with the H7 protein and the N2 protein.

Using the same example but making it a human influenza virus, the name would be A/Maryland/16/07 [H7N2]. Since it's a human virus, an animal host isn't part of the name.

two
Early History

What we know of influenza's history comes to us in bits and pieces. Assigning a specific cause to any historical epidemic comes down to, in most cases, an educated guess. Influenza's subtle ways, its commonplace symptoms, and its way of coming and going, make nailing down its past difficult.

One of the earliest possible mentions goes back to around 1250 BCE. At that time, several Greek kingdoms entered an alliance against the city-state of Troy, thought to be located in what is now northern Turkey. Disease broke out in the tenth year of the Trojan War.

The poet Homer, writing centuries later, attributed the epidemic to Apollo, the god of both health and sickness: "He attacked the mules first and the swift dogs; then he aimed his sharp arrows at the men, and struck again and again. Day and night, packed funeral pyres burned."

Some have wondered if the mysterious plague's affinity for mules and dogs suggests influenza. We know now dogs and horses catch flu. Perhaps during the Trojan War the animals picked up the disease and spread it to their Greek owners. But whether the epidemic was influenza or another disease, can never be known—and it's doubtful the Trojan War happened as Homer described it, either.

Other possible clues occasionally pop up in the historical record. The Roman writer Vitruvius described a disease that caused "cold in the windpipe, cough, pleurisy, phthisis, spitting of blood." Such illnesses, he said, were only cured "with difficulty" when they struck in cooler regions.

Influenza's tracks through human history don't definitively show up in European history until at least the medieval era. Researcher August Hirsch claimed that the earliest known outbreak of a disease identifiable as influenza took place in 1173. According to Hirsch, it was the first of ninety-four epidemics in Europe between that year and 1873.

It's clearer that thirteen pandemics of influenza have occurred since the 1500s. These true pandemics—global outbreaks—could only take place once exploration linked the Old World with the New.

Flu may have arrived in the Caribbean as early as 1493. No sooner had Christopher Columbus returned to the island of Hispaniola on his second journey than an unknown epidemic swept through its native peoples. Some historians speculate the pigs on Columbus's ships carried flu. Again, it's only a theory.

A likelier source arrived forty-six years later. Hernando de Soto amassed his first fortune working the New World slave trade. He added to it by helping the conquistador Francisco

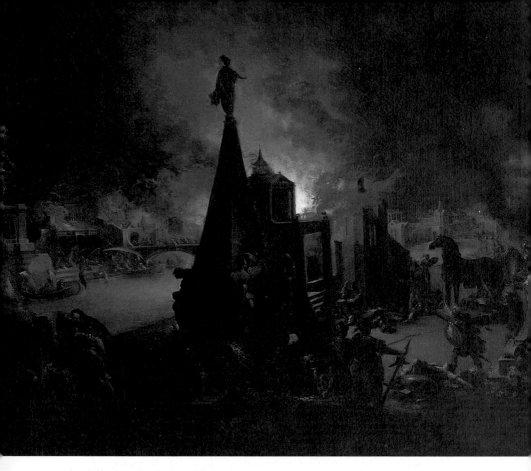

The fall of Troy, depicted by Johann Georg Trautmann (1713–1769). Some historians believe the mysterious plague described by Homer in his account of the Trojan War could have been flu.

Pizarro conquer the Inca Empire. Desiring his own command, de Soto put together his own conquistador army in 1539, intending to win gold and glory in the lands north of the Caribbean. In late spring, de Soto's force of six hundred soldiers, 220 horses—and, fatefully, three hundred pigs—landed near modern-day Tampa Bay, Florida. Spaniards on the march brought along livestock to guarantee a meat supply. Pigs had the virtue of being tough and able to keep up with the marching conquistadors.

From there, de Soto and his army set off on an expedition that spent four years torturing, enslaving, and killing Native

Americans from Florida north to the Carolinas and as far west as Texas.

Shortly after de Soto's arrival, the Timucuan, a people inhabiting northern Florida, fell ill by the thousands. Thereafter, the native peoples in the areas Soto explored suffered a tremendous decline in population, unrelated to his oppression. Archaeological finds from the period suggest that the civilizations of the time, many of them built around cities, suddenly began to dig mass graves. French explorers a hundred years later wondered at the remains of depopulated, even ruined, cities.

Whether or not the pigs brought influenza may never be known. There's no proof swine even carried flu in 1539. But we do know many European diseases had already found a way to the New World. It's reasonable to assume a virus as contagious and common as influenza crossed the Atlantic as well. That it would prosper in the crowded, urban civilizations de Soto found makes sense. Again, however, the evidence is circumstantial.

Whatever its role in the New World, influenza continued to strike Europe and Asia. "Knock-me-down fever" hit England in 1775 (and spread to its American colonies, where it caused suffering during the early part of the Revolution). From 1830 to 1833, a pandemic swept across Asia and Europe. During the worst days of the 1847 pandemic, at least a thousand people died every day in London.

Consistent with influenza's low profile, none of these visitations, nor any that came before it, left an imprint on recorded history. People suffered and died, certainly—the English and Timucuan and Chinese alike. But influenza failed to inspire the wealth of written accounts left in the wake of the Black Death in the 1340s.

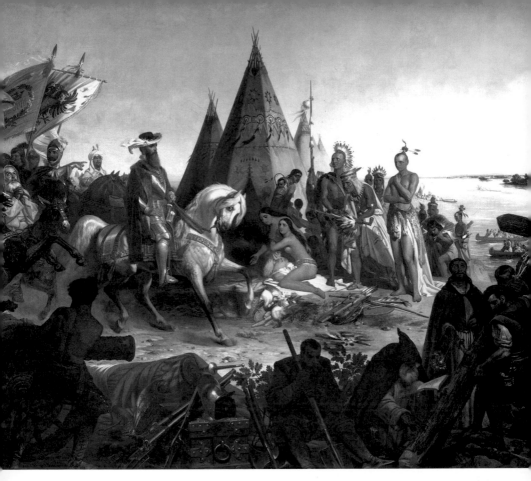

A painting of conquistador Hernando de Soto and Native Americans on the shore of the Mississippi River. Because the native population suffered a huge decline in population due to illness after his arrival, it's thought that de Soto may have brought the flu virus to North America. *(Courtesy of Architect of the Capitol)*

It wasn't until the early days of mass media that influenza became a worldwide story.

In the summer of 1889, an unusual disease broke out in the central Asian city of Bokhara, in modern-day Turkistan. The "Russian flu," as it came to be known, spread to Europe and killed an estimated 250,000 people in a matter of months.

Calling it the Russian flu was probably an inaccurate slander against Russia. Many historians believe the virus incubated in southern China. The remoteness of the Chinese interior

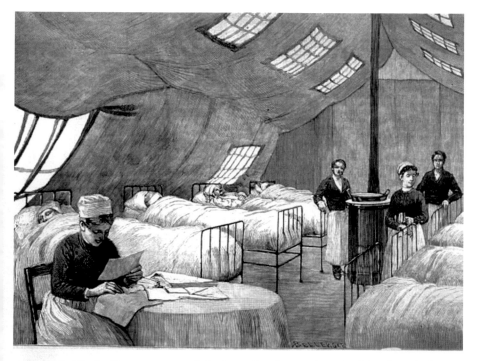

In this illustration, nurses and doctors attend to patients inside a hospital tent in France during the global flu epidemic of 1890.

and Central Asia allowed it to spread in anonymity until it exploded into prominence—and into the newspapers—in Bokhara.

Historians have since pieced together a pattern of waves of influenza occurring in subsequent years. A year after the initial Russian flu outbreak, the disease again swept around the world and caused more deaths than in 1889. In early 1892, a third, milder, wave arrived.

The Russian flu pandemic was the fourth occurring in the nineteenth century, and the worst since a deadly 1847 outbreak. Throughout the next two decades, influenza swept the world several more times, with 1900 a noteworthy year.

But it was in 1918 that a pandemic beyond all others blazed around the world. By the time it ended, the Spanish flu outbreak ranked with history's greatest medical disasters. The numbers would compare to the mortality caused by bubonic and pneumonic plague during the years of the Black Death, and by smallpox and other European diseases among New World peoples.

The difference was that the damage occurred in months, rather than in years or centuries.

Timeline of Pandemics and Other Notable Outbreaks

Pre-history Influenza crosses over from domesticated animals and infects humans.

1173 Possible year of the earliest identifiable European influenza outbreak; the disease's presence in Europe may go back to ancient times.

1500s European writings first mention major disease outbreaks definitely identifiable as influenza.

1539 Hernando de Soto leads a Spanish expedition from Florida into the North American interior; the pigs brought for food possibly introduce influenza to the Native American nations in the southeastern U.S. and Mississippi Valley.

1580 First true worldwide pandemic reaches from Europe and Asia to the New World.

1781-1782 Major pandemic in Europe, Asia, and North America; thought at the time to have begun in China.

1830-1833 Major pandemic in Europe and Asia; a related virus may have caused pandemic of 1836-37.

1847 Pandemic flu returns to Europe and the Western Hemisphere; at one point, more than 1,000 people die per week in London.

1889-	
1892	The pandemic "Russian flu" emerges in central Asia; related viruses cause death in subsequent years.
1918-	
1919	The pandemic "Spanish flu" kills 40 to 100 million people worldwide.
1957-	
1958	H2N2, a new flu subtype, causes Asian pandemic.
1968-	
1969	The "Hong Kong flu" pandemic breaks out, caused by new subtype H3N2.
1976	Death of a soldier at Fort Dix, New Jersey, leads to nationwide swine flu vaccination campaign in the U.S.
1997	Outbreak of H5N1 avian flu ("bird flu") in Hong Kong kills six people.
2003-	
2004	H5N1 avian influenza strikes across Southeast Asia.
2005	Wild birds at Lake Qinghai, China, die of H5N1; migrating waterfowl possibly carry virus to Europe, the Middle East, and Africa.
2009	Human deaths from H5N1 passed 250.

three
"Spanish Flu"

The United States entered World War I in the conflict's fourth year. Up to then, the Allies (Britain, France, Russia, and others) and the Central powers (Germany, Austria-Hungary, and others) had chewed up the lives of millions of men with weapons both tried and true (bayonets, rifles) and horrifically modern (machine-guns, artillery, poison gas). Battles raged from Belgium to Turkey, from the Italian Alps to the Baltic Coast, and across the North Atlantic, where German submarines—the U-boats—sank shipping vessels by the ton.

Epidemics had gone hand-in-hand with war since ancient times. Forcing huge numbers of human beings to camp outside for months at a time in tents, bombed-out buildings, or trenches created ideal conditions for the spread of disease. Added to that were the stresses of combat, poor food, and

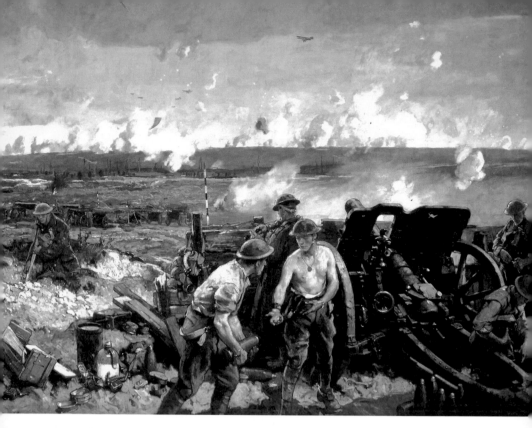

A painting of the Battle of Vimy Ridge, which took place during WWI.

the mountains of garbage and excrement created by both men and livestock.

As a rule, in wars disease killed far more soldiers than wounds. It held a six-to-one advantage over deaths in battle during the Spanish-American War. Medical experts went into the Great War aware of this grim history. But they possessed a cautious optimism. Much had changed since the wars of old.

The fifty years prior to 1918 saw the greatest advance in medical knowledge in human history. Science had buried the myths, magic, and quackery that had dominated medicine for 1,500 years. Through scientific investigation, and by the use of vaccines and sanitation, pest control and drugs, humanity had tools to fight back against disease.

The U.S. Army entered World War I determined to do whatever necessary to protect its troops from disease and infection. Military leaders educated the troops on the dangers of diarrhea, gangrene (trench foot), and typhus, as well as venereal diseases, a hazard as old as war itself. Fresh food and water became a priority. Officers stressed to soldiers the need to stay clean and dry. William Gorgas, the U.S. Army surgeon general, ordered laboratories under army supervision to manufacture vaccines and antitoxins.

In general, the military benefited from the emphasis on health. But as 1917 turned to 1918, an ever-growing population of fresh recruits packed themselves into half-finished buildings or lived in tent cities attached to training camps across the U.S. As a cold winter settled into the eastern half of the nation, measles broke out among the soldiers.

Thousands of men, especially those from rural areas, had never been exposed to the disease, and it spread rapidly. Though manageable enough in children, measles can hit adults with fever, ear infections, swelling of the brain, and convulsions. Measles-related pneumonia, however, caused the biggest problem.

Pneumonia in and of itself is a serious disease. Until 1936, it killed more Americans yearly than any other illness. Typically, the disease causes the lungs to swell with fluid. As it progresses the lung tissue becomes so saturated it cannot process oxygen. The body, starved for air, breaks down.

More than 5,700 soldiers died of measles-related pneumonia in the winter of 1917-1918. Victor Vaughan, a public health expert and founder of the University of Michigan medical school, was outraged. "How many lives were sacrificed I cannot estimate," he said. "The dangers in mobilization steps

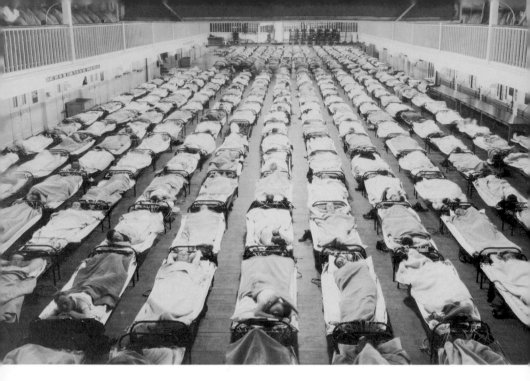

Because of the military build-up in the U.S. during WWI, most military bases were overcrowded, and the close quarters facilitated the spread of infectious illness. In this 1918 photo, naval recruits sleep in a crowded drill hall floor at a naval training station in San Francisco, California. *(Courtesy of U.S. Naval Historical Center)*

were pointed out to the proper authorities . . . but the answer was, 'The purpose of mobilization is to convert civilians into trained soldiers as quickly as possible and not to make a demonstration in preventative medicine.'"

"As quickly as possible" had become the army's unofficial motto. Speed was of the utmost importance.

President Woodrow Wilson had walked a political tightrope since the war's outbreak in 1914. Though he favored the Allies, he made no commitments, a philosophy summed up in his 1916 campaign slogan "He Kept Us Out of the War." However, after finally declaring war, he went all out. Legendary for his stubbornness, so self-possessed he seemed incapable of believing he could be wrong, Wilson intended to

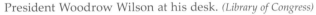

batter the Central Powers into total surrender and construct a new world order on the war's ashes.

Changing events in Europe pushed Wilson to get American troops into the field. Germany, with middling support from its Austro-Hungarian allies, had won on the eastern front. Russia's shaky communist government had settled for harsh German peace terms and left the war to tighten its hold on power.

Germany, freed from fighting in the east, hurried its troops to the western front. The plan was to overwhelm the Allied lines before American reinforcements arrived. At first the German army broke the stalemate in the trenches

President Woodrow Wilson at his desk. *(Library of Congress)*

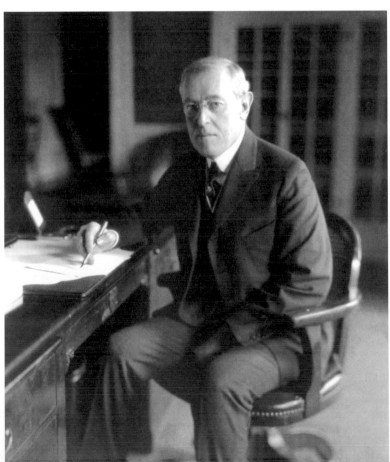

and advanced on Paris. Farther north, British troops strained to hold out along the English Channel while the exhausted Belgian and French forces neared collapse.

As that drama played out, another killer was evolving, one with power beyond that of machine guns or U-boats or poison gas.

The origins of the 1918 virus remain a mystery. Perhaps it evolved into a lethal form as it passed among soldiers packed into battlefield trenches. There is even inconclusive evidence that the virus emerged in Haskell County, Kansas, found its way to a nearby army base, and spread with soldiers on the move throughout military installations in the U.S. and Europe.

Whatever the case, the first wave of influenza arrived around March 1918.

Tens of thousands of raw recruits trained for war and army life at Camp Funston, located at Fort Riley in northeastern Kansas. Funston was at the time the second largest such camp in the U.S. On March 4, recruits began showing up sick at the camp hospital. Three weeks later, "three-day fever" had sent 1,100 men to the hospital with fever, headaches, back pain, and fatigue. Usually it passed as quickly as the nickname implied.

Soldiers from Funston, leaving for other bases or Europe, took three-day fever with them. Twenty-four of the largest army camps reported cases following the Funston outbreak. The disease turned up in cities near the camps, as well.

By early April, influenza had arrived in Brest, France, one of the major gateways for American troops headed to the battlefield. Over the next month it laid up tens of thousands of British soldiers and sailors, and made its way to Paris.

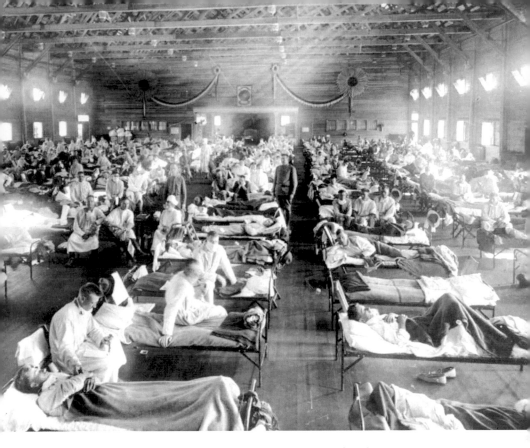

A 1918 photo of flu victims in an emergency hospital at Camp Funston. *(Courtesy of AP Images)*

At the same time, the epidemic hit the U.S. Army. In some places, six in ten soldiers were down with it—one regiment reported 90 percent of its men were sick. Most victims mended in three days. But more cases were turning into pneumonia.

The disease didn't spare the other side. "Flanders fever" ignited in the German ranks just as Germany launched a massive offensive. So many men were sick that Erich von Ludendorff, the German commander, had to postpone the attack's final phase, a move that cost his army its momentum.

Influenza had already affected military campaigns. But it had yet to make the news because the countries at war censored the press. Any report considered detrimental to morale—like an unexplained epidemic—was kept out of the papers. The average person had only a vague idea about influenza outbreaks in Europe or, for that matter, at home. Physicians and most government officials shared that ignorance.

Word began to get out, though. A respiratory virus hit San Sebastian, Spain, a popular tourist town eleven miles from the border with France. Spain was a neutral country and Spanish newspapers, free from censorship, reported on the crisis. The stories soon appeared in foreign newspapers. Readers connected the disease to the country, despite influenza's presence in other places, and nicknamed it the "Spanish flu" or "Spanish lady."

The patriotic natives of San Sebastian blamed the flu on the French. But the name *Spanish flu* stuck.

From April on, influenza spread across the European continent. It stabbed west from Spain to Portugal, reached Italy the same time it reached Paris, swept through Germany in June and into the rest of northern Europe in July and August. It reached Russia when British troops landed at Murmansk to fight communist forces. At the beginning of September, American soldiers on the same mission took it to Archangel, another Russian city. Flu immediately ran riot in Archangel's huge refugee population.

In general, the first wave of influenza, though it caused a lot of illness, didn't kill. There were exceptions. A deadlier version of the virus struck Louisville, Kentucky. Physicians noted an unusual trend. A disproportionate number of the dead victims were between age twenty and thirty-five. In the past, young adults had been least affected by "the grip" because the human immune system is at its peak at that time of our lives.

Louisville's experience turned out to be a warning.

Researchers today have a hard time discerning when the second wave replaced the first. It varied according to location. In some places the two almost overlapped. Other areas experienced a distinct separation period between the two waves. There was no first wave at all in Canada or South America.

When the second wave arrived, however, there was no doubt Spanish flu had changed. The disease now brought on ghastly symptoms, and death. Young adults would be among the most frequent victims.

On August 15, the HMS *Mantua* entered Freetown, the major port in the British colony of Sierra Leone. Two hundred of the ship's sailors had or were getting over influenza. Cases of "cattarh" appeared in Freetown shortly afterwards. On the twenty-fourth, two victims died.

As an important stop for taking on coal, Freetown received a great deal of shipping bound for important British colonies like South Africa and India. The ships that followed the *Mantua* sailed into a full-blown epidemic.

The numbers of sick and dying far surpassed the first wave statistics. On the HMS *Africa*, almost six hundred of 779 caught influenza. Fifty-one died. On the HMS *Chepstow Castle*, the figures were nine hundred of 1,150. Thirty-eight died. Another ship in port at the same time, the *Tahiti*, lost sixty-eight men en route to England and more after her arrival. Freetown and the areas nearby reported 1,072 deaths.

This mutated Spanish flu simultaneously appeared in another port city thousands of miles away: Boston.

On an average day, about 3,700 sailors bunked overnight in the barracks at Boston's Commonwealth Pier. With the war effort, however, the number swelled to more than 7,000.

Life in close quarters guaranteed the spread of any illness, let alone one as contagious as influenza. By the second week of September, 2,000 naval personnel were sick.

Thirty-five miles to the northwest of Boston sat Camp Devens. Like Camp Funston, Devens was a sprawling—and in this case, unfinished—army training center. Its camp hospital was able to handle 1,200 patients. Sick recruits had already filled all those beds in August.

On September 3, the same day Boston reported its first case, 1,400 new men arrived at Devens, bringing the in-camp population to around 45,000—10,000 over capacity.

An interior view of a crowded hospital at Camp Devens. During the month of September, 1918, flu cases at the camp swelled from one case to more than 12,000. (*Library of Congress*)

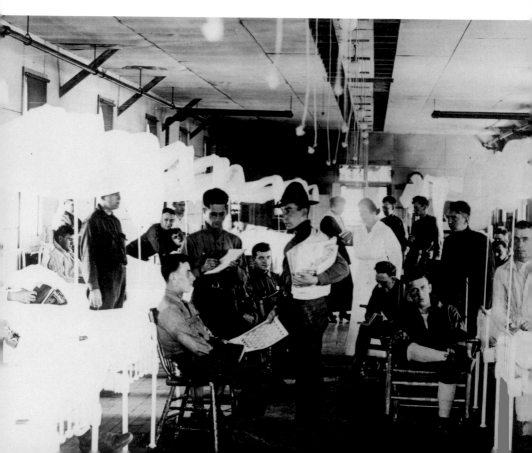

More than two dozen pneumonia cases showed up at the hospital. A dozen more soldiers, mistakenly diagnosed with meningitis, arrived on September 8.

An army report on the Devens situation described what followed as an explosion.

On September 8, the camp reported its first influenza case.

On September 10, there were 142 cases.

On September 23, there were 12,604 cases.

On September 26, the overwhelmed medical staff refused to take any more flu victims. By then, the physicians and nurses themselves had begun to die.

One of the camp doctors, Roy Grist, described "the most vicious type of Pneumonia that has ever been seen. . . . It is only a matter of hours before death comes. . . . One can stand it to see one, two or twenty men die, but to see these poor devils dropping like flies. . . ."

The dead bodies had to be stacked because there were no more coffins. Trains assigned to disposal detail took them away. Authorities converted a large barracks into a morgue.

Meanwhile, 6,000 people packed into the base hospital. The sick lay in the corridors and on porches, anywhere there was space. Blood poured out of the noses, mouths, even the ears of the living; and it leaked out of the dead when corpses were carried away. Few people remained well enough to care for the patients. And still sick soldiers streamed into the hospital, not in ones and twos but in groups.

Josie Mabel Brown, a nurse at Great Lakes Naval Station north of Chicago, recalled, "There was a man lying on the bed dying and one was lying on the floor. Another man was on a stretcher waiting for the fellow on the bed to die."

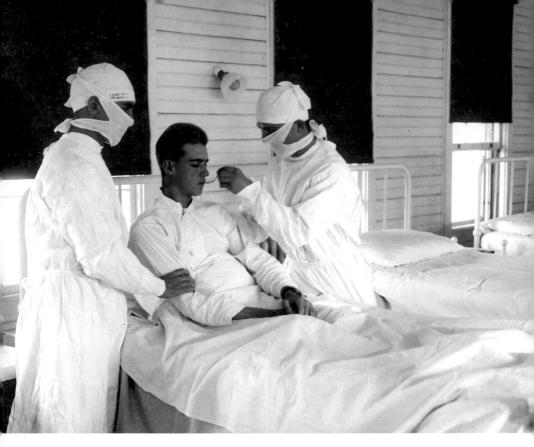

Doctors treating a flu patient at a naval hospital in New Orleans,
Louisiana, in 1918. *(Courtesy of U.S. Naval Historical Center)*

Though unsure of what the disease was, William Welch
recognized the danger it posed. Welch served in the military
as a major, but he was also the country's pre-eminent medical
expert. In an effort to slow the disease's spread, Welch asked
the army to cut off the flow of recruits to Camp Devens, and
to stop the soldiers there from leaving.

But the army leadership viewed the outbreak from another
perspective. However bad the situation at Devens—and Welch
had described a terrible scene—the army's top priority was
to fight and win the war, flu or no flu. Quarantining Devens
meant delays in the training and shipment of soldiers. Army
leaders ignored Welch's advice.

The second wave had already spread to other camps. On September 23, the army reported more than 20,000 Spanish flu cases among troops on American soil. Even this number underestimated the count.

Meanwhile, at sea, the troop transports ferrying American forces to Europe became death traps. The story of the Fifty-seventh Pioneer Infantry of Vermont is a harrowing example.

On September 27, the troops began a one-hour march. Trucks and ambulances trailed the columns of men, and picked up those too sick to go on. Once in New York City, the Fifty-seventh joined 11,000 other people (9,000 soldiers, 2,000 crew, and two hundred nurses) aboard an immense transport ship aptly named the *Leviathan*.

The sick bay was full the morning after the ship's departure. Thirty-six hours into the journey, the first flu victim died.

Groups of new patients reported sick every hour. The number soon rose past 2,000. A frightening situation became nightmarish:

> Pools of blood from severe nasal haemorrhages were scattered through the compartments, and the attendants were powerless to escape tracking through the mess, because of the narrow passages between the bunks. The decks became wet and slippery, groans and cries of the terrified added to the confusion of the applicants clamoring for treatment, and altogether a true inferno reigned supreme.

Crewmembers threw the dead overboard. In some cases, the victims went into watery graves without names, because the army had yet to give all the soldiers dog tags.

The *Leviathan* reached Brest with 1,249 aboard either too sick to go ashore or immediately moved into the camp hospital.

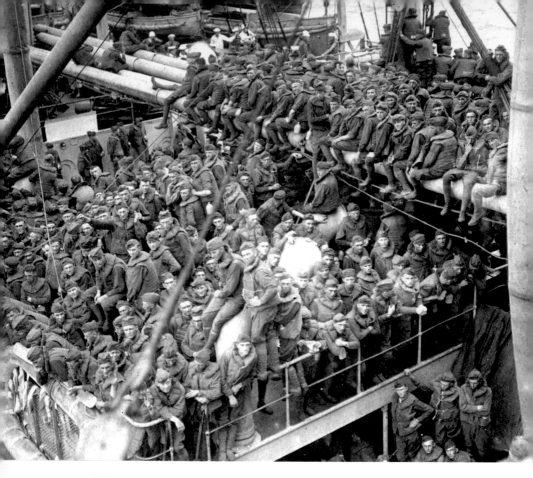

U.S. troops en route to France crowd the forward deck of the USS *Leviathan* in 1918. *(Courtesy of U.S. Naval Historical Center)*

Six hundred more fell on the road during the four-mile march to the main barracks. Civilian volunteers and members of the U.S. Navy Medical Corps followed behind to make sure they had care.

Years later, Robert J. Wallace, an army private, told his story to the historian Alfred Crosby. Wallace took ill aboard another transport, the *Briton*. With all the beds taken, Wallace, burning up with fever, lay on the ship's deck with hundreds of other men, soaked by rain and exposed to the night. Every morning, he saw medical staff take away the dead.

Finally, someone moved him to a carpeted floor below decks. When a nurse asked about his ravaged feet, he answered he'd been in the same soaked and filthy socks for twelve days.

Once on shore, Wallace saw a man in line next to him literally drop dead. Wallace, still sick, spent three days next to a kitchen stove for warmth. He lived, but lost his hair and developed an ear infection. When he returned to his unit, he realized no one knew, or cared, that he had been absent without permission.

Spanish flu peaked among naval personnel toward the end of September. It was the week of October 11 that the army finally conceded to Spanish flu. Quarantine signs went up at almost every camp. General Jack Pershing, in command of the American Expeditionary Force in Europe, received the bad news that the 78,000 new men he expected had been told to stay home. For those already in uniform, their training came to a near-standstill.

In the end, disease proved almost as deadly as the Germans. Influenza and related pneumonia killed roughly the same number of soldiers in the American Expeditionary Force—35,000—as died in combat between September 1 and November 11, the date of the armistice that ended hostilities.

Increasingly, however, Spanish flu was no longer just a military problem, if it ever had been. Every day new cases appeared, in many places at once, crossing the oceans and blazing across whole continents.

four
The Pandemic

What kind of virus was capable of killing thousands of young, healthy people and leaving thousands more racked with fatigue for weeks? Of causing such sudden and violent death? Of appearing, seemingly out of nowhere, in places thousands of miles apart? Of arriving, peaking, and dissipating in six weeks?

When it comes to Spanish flu, mystery piles on mystery. But in recent years scientists have learned a few answers.

The Spanish flu belonged to the H1N1 subtype of influenza viruses. We don't know where or how long the H1N1 circulated before 1918. But the Spanish flu did not originate in any kind of human influenza. Its genes were found in avian forms of the disease.

Terence Tumpey, a senior microbiologist at the Centers for Disease Control and a researcher of the 1918 virus, said, "[T]he 1918 virus appear[s] not to be a human/avian reassortant virus, but an avian virus that made minimal changes to infect humans directly."

Under ordinary circumstances, the average avian virus cannot latch on to human cells. The 1918 virus somehow antigenically shifted to do so. Its genetic structure appears to have undergone only slight mutation as it changed. The details of what exactly happened—and how it turned an avian flu into a killer capable of person-to-person transmission that spread worldwide—are the subject of ongoing scientific work. For example, according to a 2006 study conducted at the Armed Forces Institute of Pathology in Rockville, Maryland, a switch of ten amino acids (scattered across three proteins) separated the 1918 virus from avian viruses. At the end of 2008, a study authored by scientists at the University of Wisconsin and two Japanese institutions showed that changing a specific complex of proteins in an ordinary H1N1 virus increased its killing power. But these studies represent only pieces of what will be the final word on the disease.

Another mystery, the virus's affinity for young adults, baffled the best medical minds of the time. Under normal circumstances the eighteen-to-forty demographic is least likely to die of influenza. Today's experts still struggle to explain it. Said Dr. David Morens, a medical historian, "There are very few good theories and none of them really stand up."

Spanish flu differed from other pandemic viruses (before and since) in a number of other ways. The death rate, for instance, was between five and twenty times the norm, thanks in part to problems like pneumonia that piggybacked on the virus.

And there was one last oddity: the three waves of Spanish flu arrived on top of one another. No other pandemic we know of cycled through three waves in a matter of months. For instance, the 1889 pandemic took more than three years to run its course.

Even today, experts can only guess why any of this happened. In 1918, the long list of uncertainties—and it was longer then than now—added to the fear caused by the disease.

Though the second wave of Spanish flu caught fire in the military, civilians were also dying as early as August. Soldiers spread the disease to towns near camps and along railway routes as they headed to the coasts to disembark for Europe. Ships took it to New Orleans, to the Newport Naval Base in Rhode Island, to Seattle. It reached San Francisco by the end of September.

No American city suffered more than Philadelphia.

At the time, Philadelphia officials flattered themselves that they were ready. Hearing reports about the first wave, the local Bureau of Health put out a warning in July. The Boston outbreak made it clear Spanish flu was coming, probably sooner rather than later, if not by ship, then from one of two nearby military bases—Fort Dix in New Jersey or Fort Meade in Maryland.

A number of factors made the city vulnerable. Philadelphia had an overcrowding problem that had turned its slums into a fair approximation of an army transport ship. Newly arrived Lithuanians, Italians, Jews, Germans, and Swedes, as well as thousands of Americans, had flooded into the city to take jobs in war industries. These industries, working at maximum capacity to supply the army and the navy, attracted a lot of rail and ship traffic as well.

Philadelphia was also flamboyantly corrupt, even for an era when people considered the phrase "corrupt city government" a redundancy. Wilmer Krusen, the head of the public health department, owed his job to the political machine that ran the city. Although a physician, Krusen had no public health experience. The influenza virus at large in his city would prove far beyond his leadership talents.

Finally, there was a shortage of medical personnel. The armed forces had taken a quarter of the city's physicians and a large number of nurses. Pennsylvania Hospital couldn't find a cleaning staff, let alone doctors.

Health officials took a wait-and-see attitude when the city naval yard reported Spanish flu cases on September 11. They were confident, they said, that influenza wouldn't spread to civilians. Six days later, the navy hospital had no more room and Pennsylvania Hospital was filling up. Civilian doctors and nurses, rare enough anyway, began to get sick.

The number of cases accelerated. The first civilian (and fourteen sailors) died on September 20. Twenty people died the next day. The Board of Health suggested citizens stay warm, keep their feet dry, and avoid crowds.

The last, however, presented a problem.

The United States financed the war by selling Liberty Bonds. Those buying bonds received their money back, with interest, at a later date, while in the short term, the money paid for the war effort. Liberty Loans were offered in a party atmosphere meant to boost patriotism and, of course, the sale of bonds. Cities and towns hosted huge parades and public rallies. Salesman went house to house to sign up people.

People judged a city's patriotism by the amount of bonds it bought. Officials in Philadelphia, the home of Ben Franklin and the Liberty Bell, intended to raise millions with one of the largest events in the country.

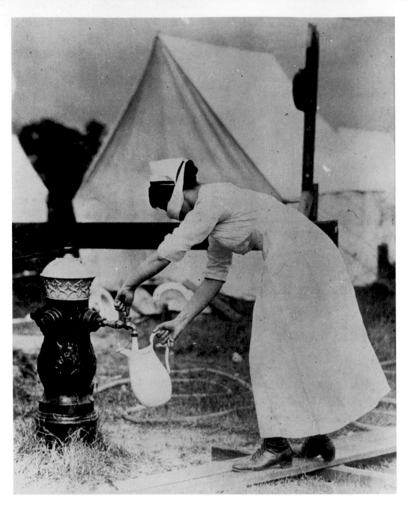

A nurse wears a mask as she fills a water pitcher outside a hospital in 1918.
During the course of the flu epidemic, many doctors and nurses also fell ill.
(Courtesy of The U.S. National Archives and Records Administration)

Fearing the crowds would cause an explosion of flu cases, physicians and infectious disease specialists begged Krusen to cancel the Liberty Loan extravaganza. The decision fell to Krusen because Philadelphia's mayor was under arrest. Krusen gave the order to go ahead with the rally.

Two hundred thousand people turned out. Politicians and celebrity speakers primed the crowd. Marching bands led patriotic sing-alongs. Anti-aircraft guns roared and planes

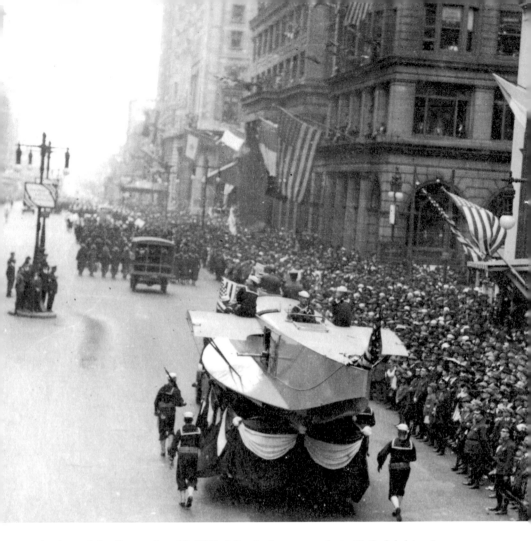

A view of the September 28, 1918, Liberty Loan parade in Philadelphia. A crowd of 200,000 turned out for this extravaganza, and forty-eight hours later Philadelphia hospitals were packed with flu patients. *(Courtesy of U.S. Naval Historical Center)*

flashed overhead. Onlookers cheered, screamed, and breathed on each other.

Forty-eight hours after the rally—the incubation period for influenza—sick Philadelphians were pouring into city hospitals. On October 1, officials reported 635 new cases of Spanish flu among civilians. Real cases probably numbered far more. Hospitals, already overcrowded, refused new patients.

Krusen took action on October 3 and ordered schools, churches, and other public places to close.

Rupert Blue, the surgeon general of the U.S., recommended similar action to public health officers across the country. "This will do much toward checking the spread of the disease," he said.

But it didn't. Two days after Krusen's order, the daily death toll in Philadelphia reached 254. On the ninth, it was 428. And it kept on rising.

The morgue, built for thirty-six bodies, had two hundred stacked like boxes. Bodies went unburied because the gravediggers were sick. Some undertakers had to keep caskets (with bodies inside) in their homes.

With so many dying, the caskets inevitably ran out. Railcars loaded with more arrived under armed guard because of the threat of theft. A streetcar company agreed to build makeshift coffins.

Desperate families iced the bodies of dead loved ones to preserve them, kept the corpses on the porch or in a spare room, or in a closet or corner, trying to ignore the sight, unable to ignore the smell. Policeman in surgical masks collected decomposing bodies in trucks or horse-drawn wagons. Priests from the local archdiocese joined them.

Civilians sometimes volunteered. Ira Thomas, catcher for the Philadelphia Athletics baseball team, taxied sick people to the hospital in his car. But Spanish flu terrified the average person. Stores closed. Hospitals ran short of volunteers. The war industries were barely able to keep producing. Flu orphans, the children of dead parents, wandered the streets.

Meanwhile, in Washington, D.C., Surgeon General Blue used $1 million in emergency funds to set up makeshift hospitals and

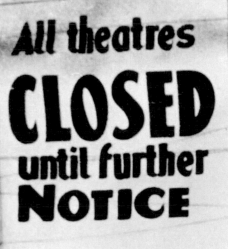

In this November 16, 1918, photo, a young boy with a flu mask stands outside a closed theater in Kansas. During the flu epidemic, many public places closed in order to stop the spread of the virus. *(Courtesy of ZUMA Press)*

soup kitchens. The U.S. Public Health Service asked retired or wounded physicians to help. For two hundred dollars a month, these doctors signed on for twenty-hour days fighting an illness no one understood.

Spanish flu cleared out immune cells from the upper respiratory system. When a victim recovered (or sometimes before), opportunistic bacteria got into the defenseless lungs and bloomed.

As a result, infections considered minor in the past turned into life-threatening pneumonia. Since there were no bacteria-fighting antibiotics in 1918—penicillin remained ten years away—bacterial pneumonia presented an enormous threat to life. Experts of the time recognized the problem. For instance, researchers at New York's Rockefeller Institute, one of the country's elite laboratories, reacted by creating a serum that fought two common pneumonia-causing bacteria. Modern-day research has confirmed bacteria's role in the pandemic. A study in 2008 showed that bacterial pneumonia, rather than the flu virus itself, killed more than 90 percent of the victims studied. Anthony S. Fauci, director of the National Institute of Allergy and Infectious Diseases, summed it up by saying, "In essence, the virus landed the first blow while bacteria delivered the knockout punch." While many kinds of bacteria invaded the lungs, the study most often found pneumococci, streptococci, and staphylococci.

Another recent invention in 1918, X-rays, helped diagnose pneumonia, while bottled oxygen assisted breathing. But both had limits. Neither was as commonplace or as safe in 1918 as they are today. Getting an X-ray meant sitting in front of radiation—even then known to cause cancer—for at least twenty minutes. Often the image was too blurry to be helpful. Regardless, hospitals packed with patients couldn't provide X-rays for everyone. The staff had a hard enough time changing the sheets.

Aspirin, so useful against minor flu symptoms, was under suspicion. Bayer had popularized the painkiller since patenting it in 1900—but Bayer had been a German company. In the patriotic atmosphere of 1918, executives at Bayer's American division spent a lot of time knocking down wild rumors that German agents laced their best-selling aspirin tablets with influenza.

Then as now, nurses provided for the day-to-day needs of patients—keeping them fed and hydrated, giving medication, monitoring sudden changes. During the Spanish flu, there were never enough nurses, not even after 1,500 answered a Red Cross call for volunteers, not even when people from teachers to dental students, from nuns to debutantes, entered the ranks. Nurses actually became more valuable than doctors. As a Boston health officer told colleagues in Maine, "Can send you all the Doctors you want but not one nurse."

Neither the spirit of volunteerism nor a medical degree prevented the flu, however. Physicians and nurses, professionals and volunteers, died in chilling numbers. And everyone involved witnessed gruesome scenes on a daily basis.

A victim able to walk might stagger into a hospital dizzy with headache and fever, his pulse racing, his throat raw and sinuses filled with fluid. Some people bled from the nose or gums. A doctor or nurse listening to a victim's chest heard a sound like crumpling paper—the lungs full of fluid and already struggling to process oxygen.

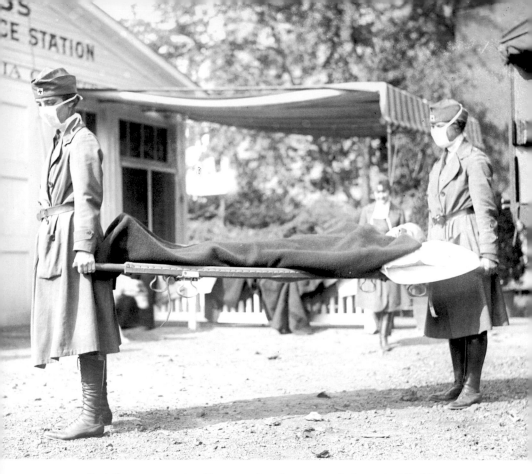

Red Cross nurses loading a patient into an ambulance in Washington, D.C., during the influenza pandemic of 1918. *(Library of Congress)*

Many patients spit up or sneezed out bloody sputum. As a case advanced, victims sometimes lost their appetite. Their voices became hoarse or they found themselves unable to speak. Those with nosebleeds lost enough blood to soak the bed linen.

The worst cases were frightful to see. Oxygen deprivation caused the lips and ears to turn blue. But it didn't stop there. Spots broke out on their faces, and then the discoloration spread. The fingers and feet turned blue and then black. Nurses learned that patients with these symptoms couldn't be saved.

Flu-related pneumonia devastated the lungs. "Some were delirious and some had their lungs punctured," said nurse Josie Mabel Brown. "Then their bodies would fill up with air. . . . You would see them with bubbles all through their arms."

Healthy lung tissue is spongy and easy to squeeze. A piece put in water would float. As a flu victim's lung filled with fluid, it became semi-solid. The hardened tissue had to work harder to exchange oxygen and carbon dioxide. In time the massive amount of fluid caused a victim to literally drown.

Scientists today continue to investigate why this happened. One theory with an increasing amount of research behind it proposes that Spanish flu caused the immune system to go into overdrive and stay there. Inflammation and the release of fluid, normally potent weapons against disease invaders,

This chart shows the mortality from the 1918 influenza pandemic in select U.S. and European cities.

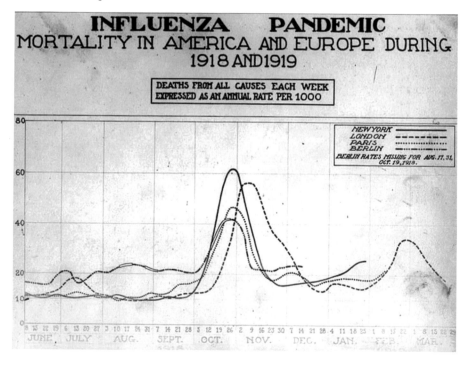

turned against a victim as the lungs swelled with liquid and ceased working.

At the same time, it seems Spanish flu provoked a massive attack by white blood cells and the other defensive mechanisms we have against viruses. It was too much. Immune cells in high amounts can be toxic, adding to the stress on a body already taxed by disease. When pushed to the limit, they attack our *healthy* cells in a berserk attempt to destroy an invader.

In fact, a severe case of Spanish flu sometimes damaged organs that ordinary influenza ignores. Herbert French, a British doctor, noted that every one of the hundred-plus victims he autopsied had bloody kidneys and, in some cases, a damaged liver. Reports of memory loss and other mental dysfunction suggest the virus sometimes affected the brain.

Middle-aged people and the elderly lack an immune system capable of mounting such an overwhelming response. One age group's immune response is robust enough, however: young adults between their late teens and age forty.

Isaac Starr was a third-year medical student at the University of Pennsylvania. In mid-September he and his classmates received a single lecture on influenza and were sent to staff an emergency hospital in a half-demolished building. Starr served as a nurse. Regular nurses and retired doctors brought back for the emergency were supposed to act as advisors. But the sick piled up so fast that "many died without having been seen by any medical attendant but me." He went on:

> When I returned to duty at 4 p.m. I found few whom I had seen before. This happened night after night. . . . The deaths

in the hospital as a whole exceeded twenty-five percent per night during the peak of the epidemic. To make room for others the bodies were being tossed from the cellar into truck, which then carted them away.

Reports tell of people who seemed healthy one moment and died hours later. Henrietta Burt played bridge into the wee hours one evening. "When we left we were all apparently well," she said. "By eight o'clock in the morning I was too ill to get out of bed, and the friend at whose house we played was dead."

Yet, for all the deaths, Spanish flu spared more than 95 percent of its victims. Some survivors took weeks to bounce back after weeks of fatigue and weight loss due to lack of appetite. Others, though, were up and around in a matter of days.

In 1918, Katherine Anne Porter, the future Pulitzer Prize-winning author, worked as a reporter in Denver. She became so ill her newspaper readied her obituary. During the illness, Porter's hair turned white, though she was only twenty-eight years old. When she recovered and left the hospital weeks later, she had lost her hair completely.

Spanish flu kept Benjamin McKilvington of Riviere Qui Barre, Alberta, in bed for three weeks. It took him three more weeks to build up enough strength to put on his clothes. When he emerged from his house, nine weeks after getting sick, McKilvington weighed eighty-four pounds—fully clothed.

By late September to early October, Spanish flu had spread to most major American cities. On September 25, eight days after sailors from Philadelphia reached Puget Sound, the disease raged in Seattle, in part because 10,000 civilians had attended a military review at a flu-stricken base.

Pages from a record book listing influenza patients in a South Beach, Washington, hospital in 1918. (*Courtesy of The U.S. National Archives and Records Administration*)

San Francisco had plenty of experience with disasters. In the first decade after 1900, it recovered from the devastating 1906 earthquake and dealt with two outbreaks of bubonic plague. Though at first the city took basic precautions against Spanish flu, San Franciscans soon gave themselves over to patriotism and allowed a series of Liberty Loan events. Flu cases boomed in the aftermath. On October 18, the city closed schools and other public places. By then basic services had started to fail. Garbage men were too sick to pick up the trash and the phone system lacked operators.

New York City reported its first influenza death on September 15. Though hard hit, New York got off easier than

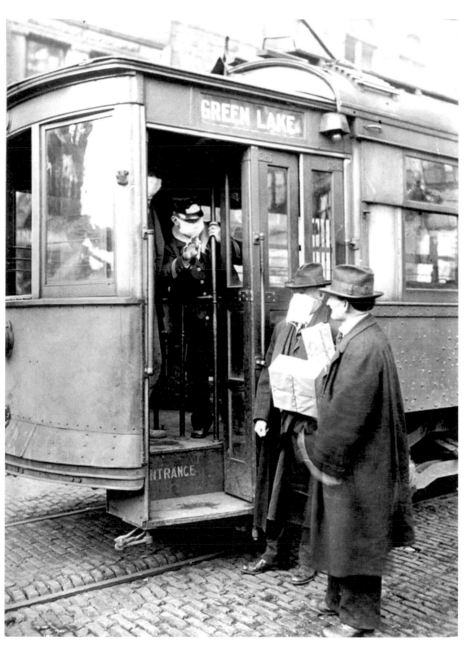

In this 1918 photo, a conductor in Seattle prevents a passenger without a flu mask from boarding his streetcar. *(Courtesy of The U.S. National Archives and Records Administration)*

Philadelphia. But it didn't get off easy. From 10 a.m. October 2 to 10 a.m. October 3—the day the *New York Times* told readers they "should not worry too much about the Spanish influenza"—city health officials counted 999 new cases and forty-eight deaths. More than two thirds of the victims were young adults.

The number continued to climb. News of Spanish flu, for days printed in the *Times'* back pages, was finally judged worthy of page one on October 5.

In towns and smaller cities, everyone knew a victim. During the epidemic's peak, even a modest-sized community might hold a dozen funerals in a single day. Thelma Trom, a twelve-year-old in Hatton, North Dakota, accompanied the local doctor on his rounds. At one point her uncle, the town's undertaker, had to keep nine caskets (and bodies) ready for burial in his garage. Most of the dead in her town were buried without a funeral.

Spanish flu's power to transmit itself allowed it to reach into the world's remote communities as well.

Teller Mission was a Native American village on Alaska's western coast. The first influenza cases showed up forty-eight hours after the arrival of a visitor from nearby Nome, the region's major town—itself infected by flu brought by boat from Seattle.

The epidemic in Teller Mission raged three weeks. Rescuers discovered twenty-five locals dead in a single igloo. The village sled dogs—half-feral animals sired by area wolves—had forced their way into another dwelling to devour the dead bodies inside. Three children turned up inside another igloo amidst frozen corpses.

Spanish flu killed all but five of the village's adults. Forty-six of Teller Mission's children ended up as orphans.

Americans didn't passively watch Spanish flu burn through the country. Early on, scientists mobilized to study the virus. National institutions like the Red Cross as well as local organizations and churches played an important role in dealing with the sick, the grief-stricken, and the orphaned.

The federal government reacted with a blitz of information. Millions of pamphlets went out to help medical practitioners and local government identify and cope with the virus. Posters appeared in offices and in public. Ads ran in the newspapers.

In the cities, public health departments churned out pamphlets in any language with a sizable constituency. Companies, needing workers on their feet, took similar steps. One mining company handed out anti-influenza literature in six languages to reach the immigrants in its workforce.

Communities took other steps as well. Closing orders, like those in Philadelphia, were popular, though two institutions—churches and taverns—often resisted.

Many local governments passed laws to minimize the chance of person-to-person spread. Ordinances mandated that masks be worn over the nose and mouth in public. In San Francisco, the Red Cross and Levi Strauss, the local blue jeans company, teamed to make and pass out masks for a dime apiece. Scenes of people wearing masks became the pandemic's iconic image. People voted in their masks, went to parties in their masks, even tried to smoke cigars in (or at least around) their masks.

Did masks prevent disease? The fabric wasn't able to filter out a particle as small as a virus. A mask of good

TREASURY DEPARTMENT
UNITED STATES PUBLIC HEALTH SERVICE

INFLUENZA

Spread by Droplets sprayed from Nose and Throat

Cover each COUGH and SNEEZE with handkerchief.

Spread by contact.

AVOID CROWDS.

If possible, WALK TO WORK.

Do not spit on floor or sidewalk.

Do not use common drinking cups and common towels.

Avoid excessive fatigue.

If taken ill, go to bed and send for a doctor.

The above applies also to colds, bronchitis, pneumonia, and tuberculosis.

2—5093

This poster issued by the U.S. Treasury Department in 1918 lists preventative measures to be taken against contracting the flu. *(Library of Congress)* construction might have stopped water droplets sneezed or coughed out by a sick person—if it was thick enough, worn correctly, and washed every day.

The American Medical Association later judged masks (and goggles) useful for doctors and others working closely with victims, but considered it too difficult to teach the public how to wear them properly.

Laws against spitting were another popular solution. At one point New York City's health commissioner said, "It does not seem to be generally known that one can receive a fine or go to jail for six months for spitting on the sidewalk." Chicago police not only arrested spitters but anyone who failed to cough or sneeze into a handkerchief.

Civilians improvised other ways of dealing with the problem:

> Our home at the time was near a chair factory, and after work many of the employees walked past our house. Occasionally, a worker would spit phlegm or tobacco on the pavement. For such occurrences, my mother always had a kettle of boiling water ready, so she could immediately scald the "damned spot" hoping to kill the unseen germs and protect my brothers from influenza.

Research suggests strategies like masks and anti-spitting ordinances reduced the number of cases and deaths if the plans worked on several levels—say, masks for people and also orders against large gatherings—and if authorities enacted preventative measures in time *and* left them in place until the danger passed.

A few cities managed to do so. Most did not. And regardless of plans, despite the number of spitters carted off to jail, whether or not firemen wore gauze masks, Spanish flu raged on. With the

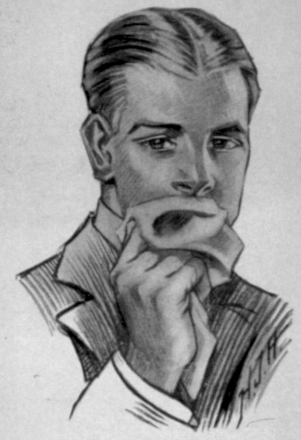

PREVENT DISEASE

CARELESS
SPITTING, COUGHING, SNEEZING,
SPREAD INFLUENZA
and TUBERCULOSIS

RENSSELAER COUNTY TUBERCULOSIS ASSOCIATION, TROY, N. Y.

A poster emphasizing the need to avoid coughing, sneezing, or spitting in public areas to prevent the spread of infectious illnesses like influenza. *(Courtesy of National Library of Medicine)*

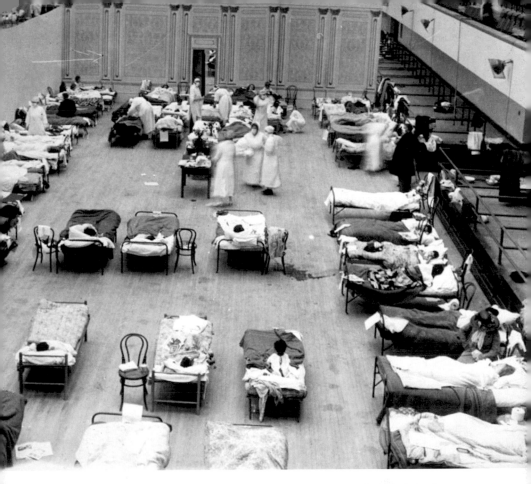

The Oakland Municipal Auditorium in use as a temporary hospital for flu victims in Oakland, California, in 1918.

medical community unable to offer much help, people took prevention into their own hands.

The revolution in medicine had pushed superstition to the fringe. Spanish flu brought it back. Victims or those fearful of becoming victims carried sulfur, a substance considered a charm against disease since ancient times. It was not unheard-of for an individual to wear a cucumber tied to the ankles or garlic around the neck. One parent buried her preschooler neck-deep in onions.

Others, opting for more modern methods, had surgeons take out their tonsils.

The tried and true also kept its place in the medicine cabinet. Vicks' VapoRub, already a popular remedy for ordinary "grip," added a shift of workers to keep up with demand. The Decatur (Indiana) *Daily Democrat* reported that the town's three-month supply had sold out in ten days.

Other sufferers rubbed goose grease on their chests and covered it with a sock, an old folk remedy for loosening a cough. Hot tea with honey was a favorite treatment, as was cayenne pepper mixed with water. Kids were given whiskey sweetened with sugar.

A doctor inoculating a patient against the Spanish flu virus during the 1918 epidemic. Doctors and scientists invented dozens of vaccines during the epidemic, but all were ineffective in warding off the flu. *(Courtesy of Hulton Archive/ Getty Images)*

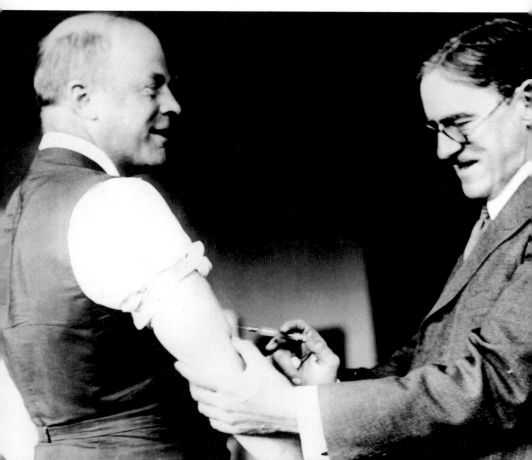

Science, though at times bad science, was popular. As the pandemic burned on, desperate physicians "vaccinated" soldiers with bacteria they mistakenly thought the cause of the disease. Doctors as well as some of America's top scientists came up with dozens of vaccines. None worked. Some victims received vaccines for typhoid and other diseases because their doctors had nothing else to give them.

Entrepreneurs saw opportunity in the crisis. "Thwart the power of the germ with Scott's Emulsion," read one ad. A well-known newspaper columnist advised his readers to use Dr. Pierce's Pleasant Pellets, a laxative, to purge toxins from the body. The makers of Grove's Tasteless Chill Tonic advised bigger doses to chase a virus more powerful than the usual "grip."

More reputable companies coiled advertising around public service. A Colgate newspaper ad prescribed the Three C's: clean mouths, clean skin, clean clothes. As it so happened, the company's famous Dental Cream (toothpaste) and Coleo Soap helped with two of the items on the list. The California Fruit Growers, meanwhile, dispensed sensible advice but also mentioned the healing properties of drinking hot lemonade every day.

Most of the rest of the world endured the pandemic without such comforts. No country, on any continent, suffered greater loss of life than India.

India, "the jewel in the crown," was the most important of Great Britain's colonies. Having survived years of famine and cholera, and a bubonic plague epidemic that killed more than 10 million people, India was hit with Spanish flu when troop ships docked in Bombay (modern Mumbai) in May or June of 1918.

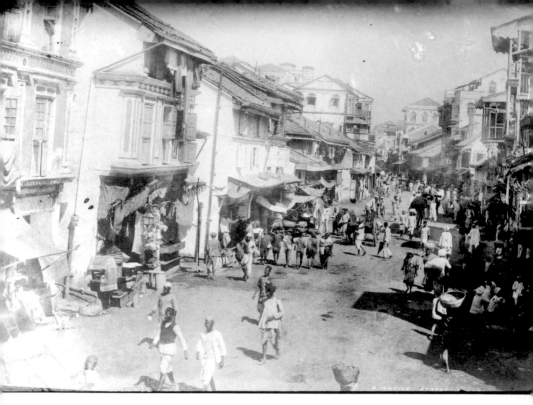

A view of Bombay, India, in 1922. India was hit especially hard during the flu pandemic, losing somewhere between 12.5 million and 18 million people. *(Library of Congress)*

Soldiers, railway workers, and others spread the disease to the rest of the country. That fall, as a food shortage picked up momentum, the lethal second wave arrived, again at Bombay. Half the population in the city and surrounding regions caught it. Since people in their twenties and thirties dominated agricultural work, there were too few workers to harvest the summer crop or plant the autumn crop.

People began to starve. Rural Indians desperate for food fled to the cities. At each train stop, rail workers took off those who had died on board. The influx of people in urban areas added to the pool of potential flu victims. One American missionary claimed influenza's death rate surpassed that of cholera or plague. In the end, Spanish flu killed somewhere between 12.5 million and 18 million Indians.

Living in remote places didn't help South Pacific islanders any more than it did Native Alaskans. Both groups may have suffered inordinately because of limited exposure to influenza viruses prior to 1918. Certainly a lack of medical care contributed.

The pandemic reached Tahiti via the *Navua*, a steamship out of San Francisco, on November 16 or 17. On December 25, the Associated Press reported that one seventh of the people in Papeete, the capital, had died.

> At the crest of Papeete burn great pyres, with the . . . sheet-covered bodies of many natives waiting to be thrown into the glowing ashes of those consumed by the flames. . . . In Papeete the victims of plague are everywhere, surrounded by the dying. Day and night, trucks rumble through the street, filled with bodies for the constantly burning pyres.

Other islands lost a fifth of the population. In western Samoa, the death rate may have soared higher. Influenza killed approximately 8,000 out of 35,000 people, and virtually everyone caught it. The pandemic only passed over nearby American Samoa because the authorities kept an airtight quarantine on the island. One in ten people on Guam perished. It devastated New Zealand's Maoris.

So it was in Brazil and Argentina, in Ghana and South Africa, in Japan and China. The official figures were staggering. And, still, huge numbers of the dead went uncounted. When the pandemic broke through Australia's quarantine in January of 1919, Spanish flu's conquest of the globe was complete.

By then the second wave had declined in most of the U.S. and Europe. A third wave, more severe than the first but less deadly than the second, rolled in around Christmastime.

Through the spring it sickened and killed hundreds of thousands more people.

President Woodrow Wilson, in Paris for talks to end the war, caught a serious case, one that may have impaired his mind. Certainly it led to behavior and decisions that baffled his aides. Once focused and decisive, Wilson found it hard to concentrate, and no longer had the strength to maintain his legendary stubbornness. He conceded several important points at the peace table and, exhausted, returned to the U.S.

The number of dead can never be known. Reliable 1918 statistics for huge parts of the world—China, Russia, most of Africa and South America—don't exist. Possibly one out of three people in the world caught Spanish flu. An estimated two or two-and-a-half percent of that number died of the disease or related pneumonia. If the percentage sounds low, remember the virus infected hundreds of millions of people. Two percent of 1 million equals 20,000 deaths.

In 1927, a study by the American Medical Association concluded 21 million people had died. Two decades later, the Nobel Prize-winning scientist Macfarlane Burnet proposed 50 to 100 million. Historians generally accept 40-50 million dead while conceding future research may revise the figure.

Even the U.S. death toll of 550,000-675,000 dead is an estimate. But, if accurate, the low number exceeds the dead in all of American wars put together, going back to the Revolution, and including Iraq and Afghanistan.

No other event in world history took so many lives in so short a time. It was, by any measure, a historic human disaster.

five
Sneezing Ferrets and Swine Flu

T he Spanish flu pandemic left almost no trail through American popular culture. The silent movies ignored it. Of the American writers of the 1920s and 1930s, only Thomas Wolfe and Katherine Anne Porter examined it in detail. It went unmentioned in histories of the Great War. The medical professionals involved skipped over it in their memoirs, and so did medical textbooks.

Scientists were the one community that maintained an interest. But they soon found that the government, like the people it represented, preferred to move on. Though measures in Congress asked for research money, little ended up being done.

Research institutions moved ahead anyway. Influenza, they knew, presented enormous challenges. For starters, there was a lack of a known cause.

Many theories were proposed during the pandemic. Not surprisingly, opposing sides in the war blamed the enemy.

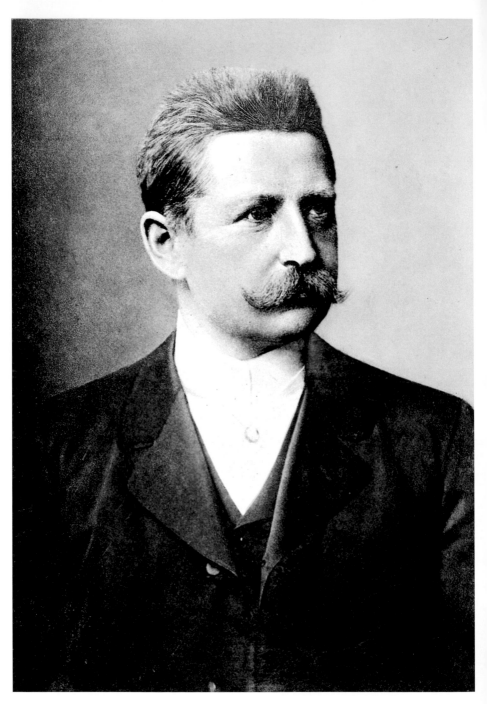

A 1906 portrait of Friedrich Johann Pfeiffer. Prior to the 1920s, most people believed that a bacterium discovered by Pfeiffer, *Hemophilus influenza*e, was responsible for influenza. *(Courtesy of Wellcome Library, London)*

Britain's naval blockade had left Germany short of food, and Germans blamed the flu on malnutrition. Americans, meanwhile, hinted at German biological warfare.

The dominant scientific theory turned out to be wrong as well.

In 1890, Friedrich Johann Pfeiffer, a scientist famous for his work on cholera, found the bacterium *Hemophilus influenzae* (or Pfeiffer's bacillus) in victims of that year's "Russian flu." Pfeiffer never claimed the bacterium caused influenza, only that it was likely. Because of his reputation, people ignored his reservations and labeled Pfeiffer's bacillus as the cause.

By the 1920s, though, the evidence pointed toward a virus as the cause. Science had for some time accepted the existence of a disease-causing agent called a virus (taken from a Latin word for *slime* or *poisonous juice*). But before 1925, when ultraviolet microscopes became available, no human being had ever seen one.

Research into another disease pointed the way to influenza. In 1926, scientists discovered the virus behind distemper, an illness fatal to dogs and related species. While searching for a vaccine, scientists learned distemper was more deadly to ferrets than to canines. Ferrets became a valued test animal.

When seasonal flu made its annual visit to Great Britain, three veterans of the distemper campaign decided to investigate it. Wilson Smith, C. H. Andrewes, and P. P. Laidlaw got samples from the throats of flu victims and infected lab animals. Ferrets again turned out to be ideal subjects. A few days after being exposed to flu, the animals had runny noses and fevers.

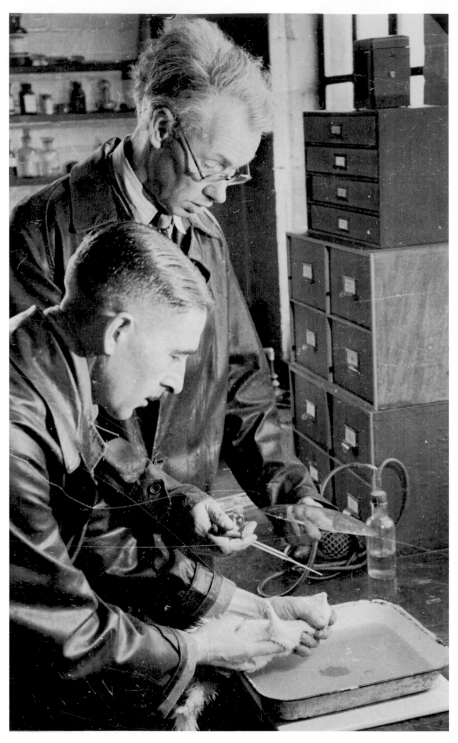

Scientists in London introduce the influenza virus into a sedated ferret as part of an experiment in this 1946 photo. *(Courtesy of Kurt Hutton/Picture Post/Getty Images)*

One day, a sick ferret sneezed in Smith's face. He felt flu symptoms come on shortly thereafter. The ferret, to his surprise, had passed the disease to him.

The virus in Smith's body became part of the experiments. He and his colleagues gave it to ferrets by dripping virus-laded liquid into the nose or putting a sick animal and healthy animal into the same cage. Twenty-six ferrets caught the disease. Autopsies showed lung damage consistent with flu. The Smith-Andrewes-Laidlaw team had isolated the virus that caused human influenza.

Other findings clarified aspects of the disease throughout the 1930s and 1940s. Scientists knew enough during World War II to produce an antiflu vaccine. As it turned out, however, the vaccine had a limited effect, because no pandemic influenza virus showed up during the war.

It came as a surprise, then, when the vaccine didn't work when a pandemic did arrive, in 1946. By then, the virus had changed into a new form through antigenic drift.

The 1946 pandemic was relatively mild. The next one, in 1958, was not. The virus emerged in southern China. Discovered in February, by June it had reached Europe and the U.S. People labeled it the Asian flu.

It turned out to be more unusual than expected. Since at least 1918, all of the human influenza viruses in circulation belonged to the H1N1 subtype. The viruses mutated and there were thousands of them, but all were H1N1s.

The Asian flu belonged to a new family, the H2N2s. Thanks to antigenic drift or, more likely, a sudden antigenic shift, the new pandemic virus was a mishmash of genetic material. Five of its genes had come from the once-dominant H1N1. An avian virus contributed three others. Scientists thought

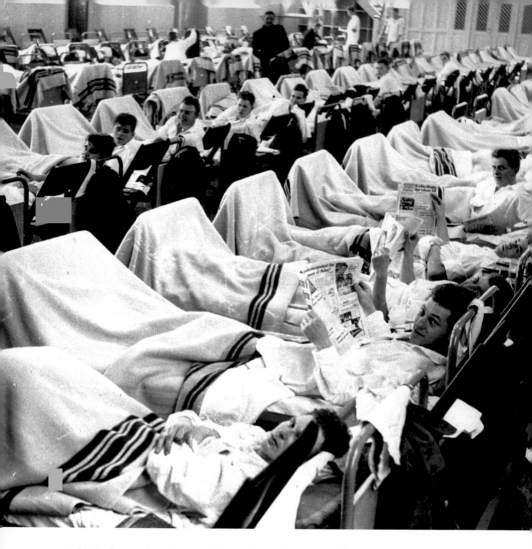

A 1957 photo of patients suffering from the Asian flu, the worst pandemic since 1918. *(Courtesy of AP Images)*

that sometime before or during early 1957, an animal—a pig or human being—caught both the H1N1 human and an avian H2N2 virus at the same time and hosted a reassortment.

The resulting influenza was extraordinarily dangerous. Being partially a human virus meant that it could spread person-to-person. At the same time, no human being had immunity to its avian genes. Once a person caught Asian flu, his or her immune system had no idea how to fight it.

Fearing a repeat of 1918, American public health officials asked President Dwight Eisenhower for a nationwide vaccination campaign. The administration, however, preferred to leave the response to the business sector and individual citizens.

Crates of Asian flu vaccine being rushed to hospitals by helicopter in 1957. During the 1957-58 pandemic, 45 million people caught the flu in the U.S. *(Courtesy of Walter Sanders/Time Life Pictures/Getty Images)*

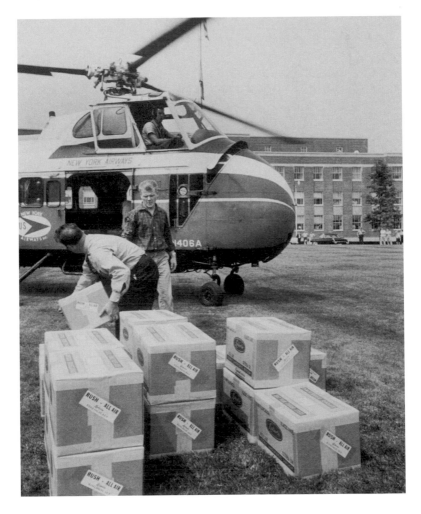

The Asian flu turned out to be the worse pandemic since 1918. Worldwide deaths may have reached 2 million. In the U.S., 45 million people caught the flu. Between 70,000 and 80,000 died.

A decade later, in 1968, pandemic flu returned. In July, the so-called Hong Kong flu broke out in southeast China. The new virus was also the product of a reassortment, this time between an H2N2 and a virus from ducks. Thereafter, the new family of viruses, subtype H3N2, dominated. The virus's descendants, also H3N2s, cause human influenza today.

Hong Kong flu reached the U.S. and Japan at the end of 1968. Because the virus had inherited part of its genetic structure from the Asian flu, people who had caught the 1957 virus had partial immunity.

Hong Kong flu hit Europe harder than the U.S. Deaths in Great Britain numbered about 30,000, only 4,000 fewer than the 34,000 who died out of the larger American population.

Influenza's next appearance on the world stage would gather much greater attention, despite the fact that the death toll equaled exactly one person.

As the U.S. prepared to celebrate its bicentennial, the summer of 1976 became the summer of swine flu.

The swine flu story really began during the Spanish flu pandemic. On September 30, 1918, an unknown flulike virus struck the pigs at the annual Cedar Rapids Swine Show in Cedar Rapids, Iowa. The disease caused fever and runny noses in many animals, but in the worst cases, the pigs died in less than two days.

After the show ended, farmers and their swine returned to farms across the Midwest. The disease traveled with them.

Throughout the fall and early winter, the mystery virus killed thousands of pigs.

J. S. Koen, a government inspector, investigated the disease and coined the term "swine influenza" to describe it. He insisted it acted like influenza and looked like influenza, and that there was evidence humans and swine caught it from each other. "I believe I have as much to support this diagnosis in pigs as the physicians have to support a similar diagnosis in man," he said.

Swine flu flared up in pigs every winter after 1918. It arrived with the season's cold and wet, sickened pigs for three months, and went away until the next year. Farmers and the pork industry accepted the disease as one more aspect of their business, and, as technology allowed, developed vaccines to protect their herds.

Then, in February 1976, an unusual case of swine flu surfaced—not on a pig farm, but at Fort Dix, New Jersey.

Private David Lewis reported sick on February 4 with fever, fatigue, and nausea. Influenza—the ordinary human kind—was going around the base. A medical officer told Lewis to recover in his quarters for forty-eight hours.

Lewis, eager to prove himself, insisted on going on that night's hike with his unit. During the night he collapsed. He died hours later at the base hospital. Doctors blamed his death on influenza complicated by pneumonia.

The base's medical commander sent throat samples from Lewis and eighteen other sick recruits to the New Jersey Department of Public Health. Tests revealed that eleven had the ordinary human influenza going around that year.

The rest had something unrecognizable. New Jersey officials sent those samples to the Centers for Disease Control (CDC) in Atlanta.

The CDC needed a week to match it to a known influenza virus. Lewis and the others had swine flu. In fact, the virus appeared to be almost identical to a swine influenza virus isolated in the 1930s. To add to the disquiet, it belonged to the H1N1 subtype, the family that included the Spanish flu.

The finding set off alarms. Had Spanish flu circulated in swine all those years? Or, if not the exact virus, something similar? If so, had it infected Lewis? Had he or someone else spread it to others?

A follow-up investigation raised more fears. Neither Lewis nor the other men infected with the same virus had any exposure to pigs. That suggested their influenza had passed from an unknown person to Lewis and the others.

David Sencer, the director of the CDC, organized a meeting of the country's leading public health scientists. The attendees discussed various aspects of the Fort Dix virus and the threat it posed. Despite many unanswered questions, the scientists agreed to go ahead with researching a vaccine for the Fort Dix virus.

"We have the technology, we have the evidence of transmission," Sencer said. "It would be irresponsible to do anything else except develop a vaccine."

Public health experts felt they had reason to worry. At the time, it was widely accepted that pandemics took place every eleven years or so. A postwar pandemic had hit in 1946, the Asian Flu in 1957, and the Hong Kong Flu in 1968. Though only eight years had passed since then, a sped-up timetable for the next pandemic virus wasn't out of the question, given influenza's unpredictability.

Then there was the public. Americans, by and large, ignored advice to get the annual flu vaccination. Even in 1968, the year of a serious virus, just over 10 percent bothered. Physicians had as little interest. If the Fort Dix virus could lead to a disaster like 1918, officials needed as much time as possible to convince people they needed the vaccine.

In this 1976 photograph, Gary Noble discusses the swine flu virus with David Sencer (right) at the Centers for Disease Control headquarters in Atlanta, Georgia. *(Courtesy of Centers for Disease Control and Prevention)*

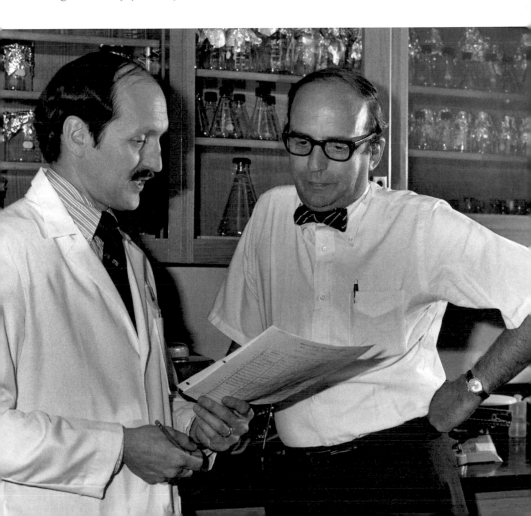

The experts, like all scientists cautious by nature, recognized there were too many unanswered questions to definitely predict a pandemic. So they played the percentages. Certain indications were that the Fort Dix virus had the *potential* to become lethal and contagious. As one expert put it, "[T]he possibility of a swine flu outbreak in the future could not be disproved. What could not be disproved must be allowed for."

Another, years later, said, "Better a vaccine without an epidemic than an epidemic without a vaccine."

A majority of the experts wanted to ask the government to fund a nationwide vaccination campaign.

A few dissenters took a more cautious approach. Better, they said, to stockpile vaccine and wait to see if a pandemic developed.

The first group countered that it would be too difficult to get out 200 million doses of vaccine once the pandemic started. Clinics had to be organized, staff assigned. That took time. "By the time we vaccinated everyone under the stockpile theory," one expert recalled, "millions would have had ample opportunity to catch the flu."

Furthermore, for a vaccine to have maximum effect, people needed a shot a few weeks before flu arrived, to give the immune system time to create antibodies against it.

CDC director Sencer sent his superiors a report laying out the facts and proposing options. One was to do nothing. But the favored proposal asked for $134 million to create and distribute a swine flu vaccine to the American public.

A group of experts met with President Gerald Ford on March 24. The gathering included Jonas Salk and Albert Sabin, heroes of the polio vaccination campaign in the 1950s,

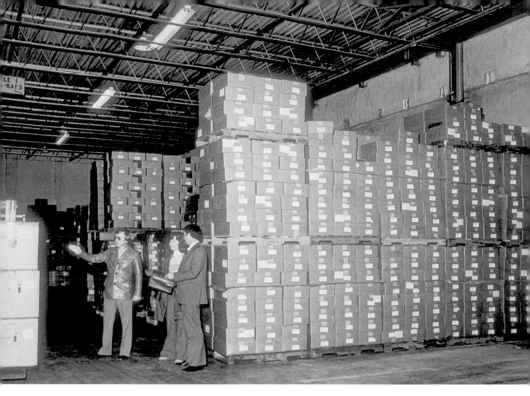

Stockpiled boxes of swine flu vaccine in a warehouse in 1976. *(Courtesy of Centers for Disease Control and Prevention)*

and two of the best-known scientists in the country. Also there were physicians, public health officials, scientists, politicians, and drug industry representatives.

During the meeting, Ford asked some of the people present if the nation faced a swine flu epidemic, and if mass vaccination was necessary. No one responded, not even those who had voiced reservations before. Ford offered to hear out any doubts in the privacy of his office. Not a single person took him up on it.

That evening, he drafted Salk and Sabin to stand beside him as he announced the vaccination campaign to the nation. He declared his intention to ask Congress for $135 million to inoculate every American citizen.

Once politicians got involved, the vocabulary scientists used—words like "if," "possibility, "theoretically"—was deleted from the public discussion. Sencer's memo had underplayed comparisons to 1918 for fear of exaggerating the threat. But others in the government brought up Spanish flu time and again. From then on, the 1918 pandemic became the reference point, the event to be avoided at all costs, even though the scientific community was uneasy with the comparison. When Ford signed the bill appropriating money for the campaign, he flatly (and wrongly) said the swine flu virus at Fort Dix and the Spanish flu were the same.

The possibility of a pandemic, once an *if*, was increasingly considered a matter of *when*.

Critics, meanwhile, accused the CDC and government of rushing into the vaccination campaign. Many advocated for the stockpile idea. Albert Sabin, an influential voice, came to favor it. A number of insiders also turned against the program. A few staffers at the CDC were opposed. Ford's own advisors, while not against it, worried about how swine flu might affect the president's fall re-election campaign.

Opposition to vaccination grew throughout the spring and summer. Then things began to go wrong with the vaccine.

One of the manufacturers, Parke-Davis, used the wrong virus. Two million doses had to be destroyed.

As tests continued, it became clear the vaccine didn't work well in children. The journal *Science* reported that "none of the vaccines provided sufficient protection without causing unacceptable side effects."

The Pharmaceutical Manufacturers Association, a lobbying group for drug companies, presented the Ford Administration with another headache. Drug manufacturers refused to rush a swine flu vaccine to market unless the government assumed legal responsibility for anyone harmed by the product. This meant that taxpayers would pay the penalties if the vaccine hurt or killed people.

That touched off more debate. Critics accused the companies of shirking their responsibilities to the public good. Manufacturers replied that their insurers refused to cover anything to do with swine flu, leaving companies on their own financially.

Both houses of Congress went back and forth over the issue. Opinion seemed to go against the manufacturers. That, in turn, threatened to touch off a crisis, because the manufacturers continued to refuse to produce vaccine without legal protection.

An incident in Philadelphia broke the deadlock.

On August 2, the media reported an unidentified illness in Philadelphia. Approximately 150 cases and twenty deaths were related to an outbreak at a hotel hosting an American Legion convention in late July. At a glance the so-called Legionnaire's Disease, a respiratory illness, resembled influenza. Some thought the dreaded swine flu had arrived at last.

Three days after the first reports, on August 5, the CDC ruled out swine flu as the cause of Legionnaire's Disease. But the inability of the investigators to come up with another cause kept the story in the news. The scare, meanwhile, gave the vaccination campaign new momentum.

The National Swine Flu Immunization Program became law on August 12. The government, and through the government the taxpayers, assumed the legal risks, as the drug companies had demanded. Vaccinations began October 1.

The campaign hit its next snag ten days later.

The October 11 edition of the Pittsburgh *Post-Gazette* reported the deaths of two local people. Both were over age seventy. Both had died within a short time of receiving the swine flu vaccine.

The deaths became a national story. President Ford, appearing on the *CBS Evening News*, cautioned against drawing any conclusions. The next day, he received his flu shot, as did his family.

Forty million Americans would get a swine flu shot by mid-December. By then, however, the vaccination campaign was on its last legs. Another mysterious illness had appeared. And this one seemed to have a definite connection to the vaccine.

An elderly woman receives a vaccination by a public health worker during the nationwide swine flu vaccination campaign in 1976. *(Courtesy of Centers for Disease Control and Prevention)*

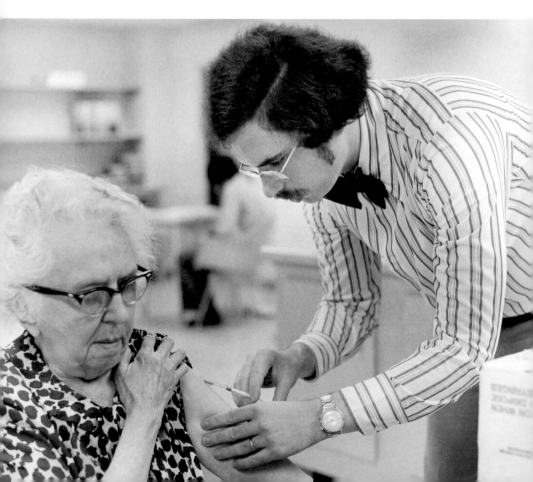

In mid-November, a Minnesota doctor reported a case of a rare disorder, Guillain-Barré (ghee-yan bah-ray) syndrome, to health officials. Guillain-Barré syndrome caused a victim's immune system to attack the peripheral nervous system. A case often started with fatigue and tingling in the legs. As it intensified, the arms and upper torso were also affected. Severe cases caused paralysis. Those patients often needed machine-aided respiration because the chest muscle couldn't move to breathe.

Most Guillain-Barré patients recovered. In some cases, though, paralysis lasted weeks or months, sometimes up to three years. There were rare instances of permanent paralysis or death.

On December 14, a CDC press release said the agency had found fifty-four cases of Guillain-Barré syndrome that had appeared following a swine flu shot. Sencer, the CDC director, halted the campaign the next day. By the end of the year, 526 Guillain-Barré cases had appeared. Not all the sick people had been vaccinated. But 257 had. Both numbers more than doubled in the next month.

More than 4,100 lawsuits were filed. By 1993, the swine flu vaccination campaign had cost taxpayers almost $93 million in settlements and awards.

The virus behind the trouble remains unexplained. No one knows who brought it to Fort Dix. No one knows why Private Lewis, alone of those infected, died. No one knows why the vaccine worked best in people born before 1957, and was ineffective in everyone else. Nor is anyone sure where swine flu went. Though it had emerged in modern times, in the spotlight of the mass media, and on the watch of an established, experienced scientific community, swine flu vanished—another of influenza's unsolved mysteries.

Timeline of early scientific progress

1892 Friedrich Johann Pfeiffer proposes bacterium *Hemophilus influenzae* (Pfeiffer's bacillus) as cause of influenza.

1920s Tests show Pfeiffer's bacillus not the cause.

1933 Wilson Smith, C. H. Andrewes, and P. P. Laidlaw isolate human influenza virus.

1940 Thomas Francis isolates influenza B virus.

1941 Discovery of the hemagglutinin (H) protein.

1943 First effective influenza vaccine developed.

1946-1947 Vaccine fails against mild pandemic.

1957-1958 Asian flu pandemic kills between 70,000 and 80,000 Americans.

1963 Development of amantadine, the first anti-influenza medicine.

1968-1969 Effective vaccine created for Hong Kong flu pandemic, but most Americans pass on getting shots; U.S. death toll is around 30,000.

six

H5N1

On May 21, 1997, Lam Hoi-ka, a three-year-old Hong Kong boy, died of a severe respiratory illness. Before taking ill, he'd been healthy, active—a normal preschooler.

He had gotten sick twelve days before with a fever and sore throat. Congested lungs and then breathing problems followed. Pneumonia soon strained the boy's lungs. Then Reye's syndrome, a rare disorder, caused excess fluid to flood his head. His brain, too heavy, descended into the brain stem, the center for regulating unconscious physical activity like breathing and heartbeat. The boy mentally deteriorated. Numerous organs—lungs, liver, kidneys—started to fail. Before he died, his blood no longer clotted.

A Hong Kong laboratory discovered influenza virus in fluid swabbed from the boy's throat. At first the technicians figured the virus would belong to the H3N2 subtype, the family of viruses that had dominated human influenza since the 1960s. But they found no match, regardless of how many tests they ran.

The lab sent freeze-dried samples of the virus to major influenza research facilities in London, Atlanta (the Centers for Disease Control), and the Netherlands. These places had far more extensive collections of viruses to test against—whole libraries containing thousands of strains.

In the Netherlands, a flu expert named Jan de Jong started work. He tested the sample against human viruses, swine viruses, and others rarely seen anymore. The sample didn't have to show a perfect match. Researchers recognize a new virus might only partially resemble something they've seen before. The degree it matches depends on how closely the two are related.

The Hong Kong sample appeared unrelated to anything. De Jong forwarded it to his country's major influenza center. There, scientists had access to even more kinds of flu. It took a week, but they found a match.

The boy had contracted a kind of flu in the H5N1 family. H5N1 viruses were thought to be avian influenza—bird flu. In 1997, scientists believed avian flu viruses couldn't spread to human beings without first reassorting with a mammalian virus. (This has since been disproved.) Proteins on an avian flu virus weren't supposed to latch onto human cells—they're too different from the cells inside birds. This lack of compatibility is part of the species barrier that protects us from animal viruses (and vice versa).

That an avian virus could bind to human cells—that an H5N1 had jumped the species barrier—stunned the researchers.

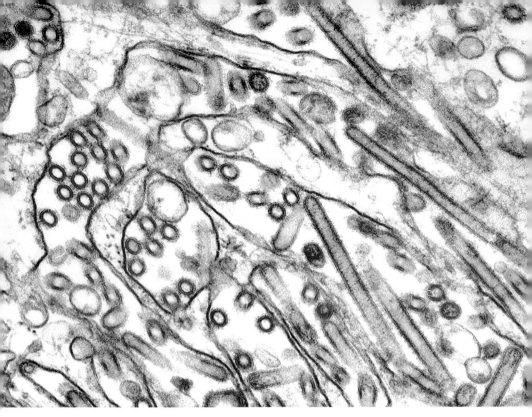

A transmission electron micrograph image of H5N1 flu viruses (seen in gold).
(Courtesy of Centers for Disease Control and Prevention)

An H5N1 virus able to infect humans presented two dangers.

First, the human immune system had never seen an H5N1. For that reason, it threatened every person, everywhere.

Second, once the virus got past the species barrier, it might mutate to become better at infecting humans and spreading between them. From that point on, an epidemic—even a pandemic—became increasingly likely.

As a rule, scientists distrust any result that's too dramatic. Finding a human being infected with an H5N1, something that had never happened, qualified. Hong Kong authorities, aided by scientists from several outside countries, launched an investigation to see if Lam Hoi-ka really died of bird flu and, if so, where he got it.

Investigators checked whether an avian influenza had contaminated the boy's samples in the laboratory. They asked if the boy had spent time on poultry farms in rural areas near the city, or if the family or anyone near their house kept birds in the backyard; if they knew anyone who had suffered from influenza; or if they had gone to one of the city markets offering live birds for sale.

All the answers were negative.

Having checked the family off the list, the investigators turned to the staff and students at the boys' preschool. The only clue was that the boys' class had played with baby chickens and baby ducks brought in as pets. Most of the birds had died shortly afterward. Researchers tested particles from the classroom and the school grounds but turned up no sign of a flu virus.

Unable to determine how the boy caught H5N1, the investigators next looked into whether he'd spread it to others. Four people came up positive. None of them became seriously ill, however. Nor did any of them come from those around the child the most—his family. Surprisingly, however, five people with no link to the boy also tested positive. All had jobs in the poultry industry. They, too, were infected, but showing no signs of illness.

The international experts, satisfied the virus hadn't spread, left Hong Kong.

Avian influenza returned in November.

On November 6, another young boy, this one two years old, went to the hospital with flu symptoms. Tests showed he had the H5N1 virus. Nonetheless, he got better in two days and went home. Then, on November 17, an adult man, aged thirty-seven, spent a week in the hospital with more severe avian flu symptoms.

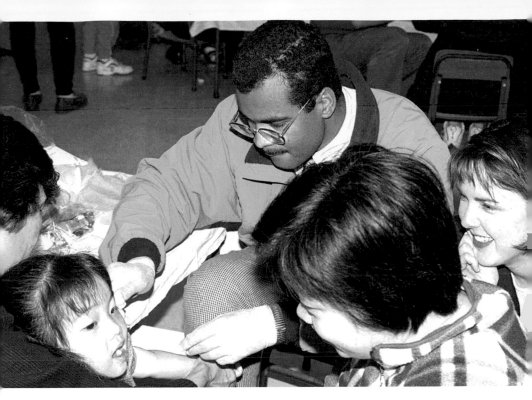

A doctor from the Centers for Disease Control takes a blood sample from a classmate of one of the children who contracted bird flu in Hong Kong in 1997. *(Courtesy of AP Images)*

Throughout December new cases were reported, as were deaths from the virus. Autopsies on two of the dead victims showed extensive damage to the lungs, liver, and kidneys, and terrible swelling in the brain. It appeared much of this damage wasn't done by influenza, but by an out-of-control immune system.

Scientists worried that many H5N1 cases, perhaps most, were going undiagnosed, either because a sick person didn't come to the hospital to be tested, or because he or she was asymptomatic. Both kinds of victim would be contagious and might fuel an explosive outbreak if the virus spread from person-to-person.

Another team of experts hurried to Hong Kong. There they joined local scientists scrambling to find the virus's source.

Money from Hong Kong institutions and the U.S. government helped set up a special laboratory to keep the virus contained. Other labs were brought up to higher security standards. The team's leaders sent out a call for supplies and technicians, and asked virologists to come to Hong Kong.

The questions asked the previous summer came up again. Did the H5N1 spread person-to-person? Could it cause a pandemic? Close to thirty years had passed since the last one. Experts considered the world overdue for another. Was this it? Avian flu might cause a 1918-like disaster. If that scenario was playing out, the virus had to be stopped before it escaped Asia and swept over the world.

Investigators found the flu victims had one thing in common. They had visited settings where poultry was present. With that in mind, scientists turned their attention to Hong Kong's birds.

There had been news of sick birds in the early part of the year. One farmer described birds suffocating, turning dark green and black, and keeling over. In other cases, chickens lost appetite and coordination, coughed and sneezed, and had trouble laying eggs. The dead birds' insides looked like something that had come out of a blender.

Investigators were also aware of Hong Kong's proximity to China. All but one of the known pandemics had been traced to the country's south in general, and Guangdong, the province attached to Hong Kong, in particular. Geese had died of a flulike illness the previous year.

And 80 percent of Hong Kong's chickens came from farms in China.

Before arrival, a bird might live for several days in close quarters with other birds. Once in the city, many thousands

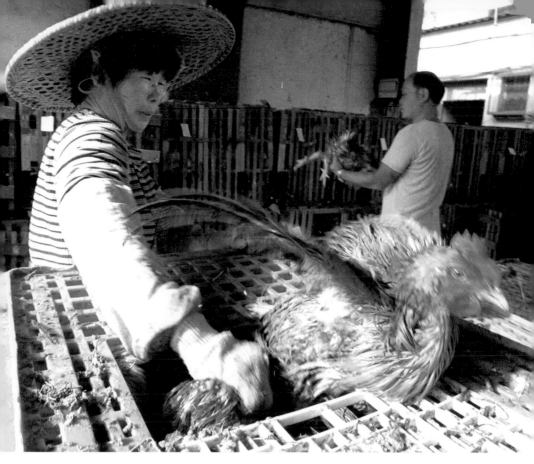

A 1997 photo of a worker catching chickens at a poultry market in Hong Kong. *(Courtesy of AP Images)*

of chickens were sold in the "wet markets." At a wet market, the butchers killed the birds (and many other animals) right in front of the customers, as per Chinese custom. Hygiene was not a high priority. Waste and blood sometimes clung to the dead bird, the butcher, the customer, or the cages stacked nearby.

As it turned out, tests on fecal matter taken in the wet markets showed 20 percent of the chickens carried H5N1. Investigators soon traced the chickens to farms in mainland China.

"The important question to me is: how is the virus getting across to humans?" Kennedy Shortridge, at the time head of

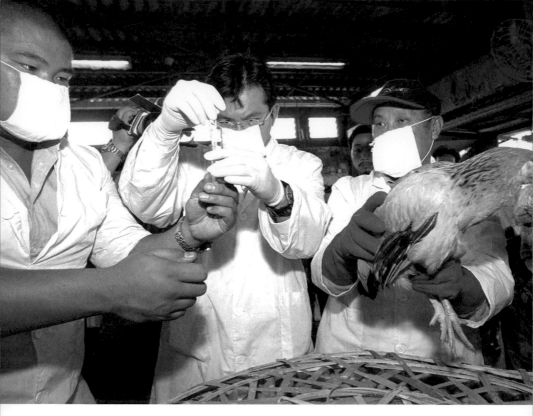

Government veterinary officers taking samples of chicken feces at a Hong Kong poultry market in 1997. *(Courtesy of AP Images)*

the University of Hong Kong's Department of Microbiology, told the *New York Times*. "The second important question is: will this virus undergo any transformation that will allow it to infect humans and cause an epidemic or a pandemic?"

Scientists on the scene worried about antigenic shift. That seemed a particular danger because this new outbreak had come in December, the start of Hong Kong's annual flu season. Thousands of people were sniffling and coughing with that year's ordinary human flu. If one of them also caught the H5N1, he or she could be, in theory, the mixing bowl for a lethal reassorted virus.

In the meantime, people in Hong Kong, hearing rumors of a possible deadly flu, edged closer to panic. Frightened pet

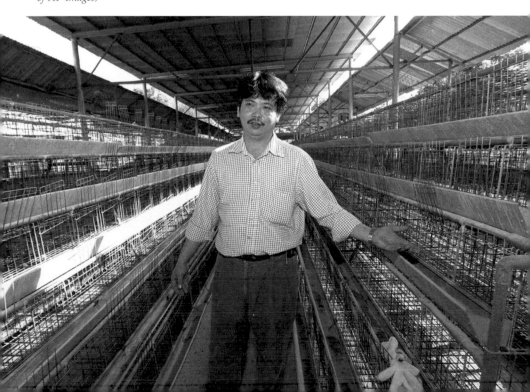

owners left pigeons and cockatoos with animal shelters. Hong Kong's thirty-plus newspapers ran increasingly frightening stories. Hospitals, unable to cope with the crush of worried people during office hours, screened for influenza twenty-four hours a day.

The investigators were confident the H5N1 virus came from chickens. Faced with the possibility it might mutate into something worse, they suggested slaughtering every chicken, duck, quail, and pigeon in Hong Kong.

Poultry sellers protested, as expected. But on the morning of December 29, workers fanned out among a thousand businesses and across 160 farms. Birds were gassed, disinfected, and buried in landfills, or had their throats cut before

A Hong Kong chicken farmer walks through his empty chicken coop in 1998. After an outbreak of bird flu, the Hong Kong government decided to slaughter all chickens in the region in an attempt to prevent a bird flu epidemic. *(Courtesy of AP Images)*

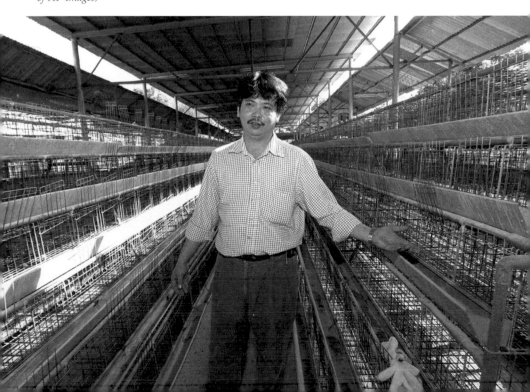

being disposed of. There were so many to kill that the government had to pull dogcatchers and gardeners from their duties to help.

It took four days to slaughter an estimated 1.2 million chickens and 400,000 other birds. Hong Kong closed markets to live birds until February (May for ducks and geese) and passed new regulations. Hard-to-clean wooden cages were out, replaced by plastic. Authorities quarantined birds coming in from China to make sure none carried H5N1; China tested on their side as well. Each species of bird was kept separate from the others.

The slaughter appeared to work. The last human H5N1 case appeared on December 28.

Experts knew the virus might return. But they took comfort in the fact that victims caught the H5N1 due to exposure to birds. The alternative—that it was contagious between human beings—would have been a step toward a pandemic.

But, even though this bird flu wasn't supposed to infect human beings and there was no previous record of a human being ever catching it, eighteen people were infected. Six died, putting the death rate at a staggering 33 percent. Who it killed was just as troubling. Three of the dead were young adults. And every influenza researcher in the world knew the pattern matched one last seen in 1918.

The occurrence shared something else with the Spanish flu. The H5N1 hadn't needed to reassort with a human virus before crossing the species barrier. At the time, that went against a long-held theory. Some years later, Jeffrey Taubenberger, at the Armed Forces Institute of Pathology in Maryland, discovered that the 1918 virus was also avian. In

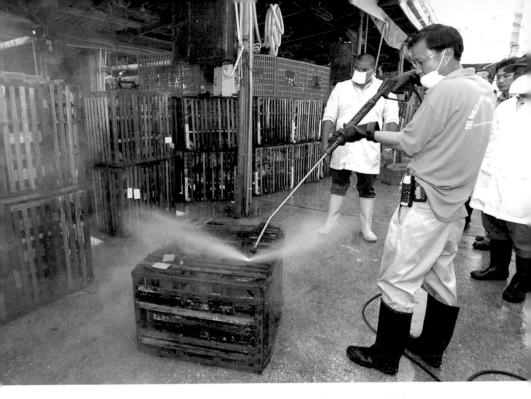

A Hong Kong government employee spraying disinfectant on chicken cages in 1997. *(Courtesy of AP Images)*

hindsight, Hong Kong looked like a close call with disaster.

After Hong Kong, the World Health Organization, the CDC, and other public health institutions strengthened the global system for monitoring influenza. New labs were built. The international scientific community encouraged China to contribute. Other Asian countries like Vietnam tracked and reported outbreaks for the first time.

For five years, H5N1 left humanity alone. But it continued to spread through birds. In a rare result among flu viruses, it killed them. An animal's system simply crashed, assaulted all over by the invading disease.

The H5N1 returned to Hong Kong in 2002, this time in the city's beloved exotic and wild bird population. Wild ducks and geese, egrets and herons, even the flamingoes, started to die.

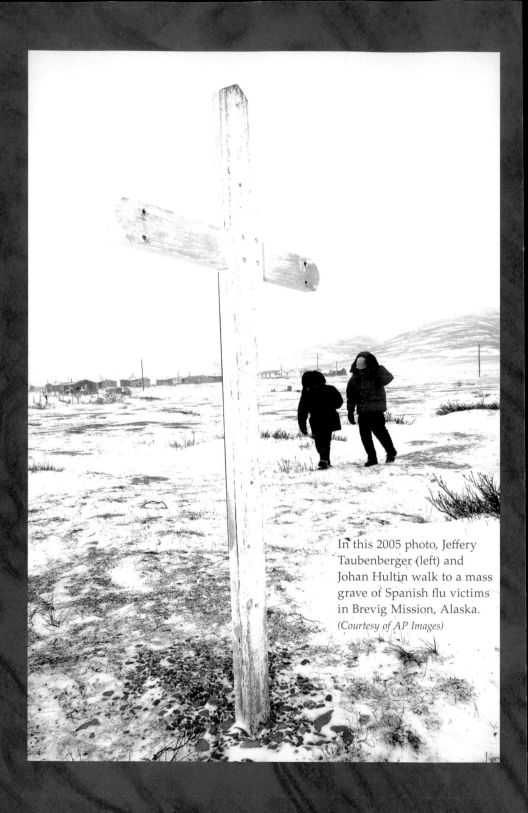

In this 2005 photo, Jeffery Taubenberger (left) and Johan Hultin walk to a mass grave of Spanish flu victims in Brevig Mission, Alaska.
(Courtesy of AP Images)

"It suggests the virus is not necessarily confined to that park in Hong Kong, because it was found in free-roaming waterfowl," said Klaus Stöhr, the director of the WHO's influenza program. The statement turned out to be prophetic.

Two months later, bird flu reappeared in humans to the north, in China. A seven-year-old girl in Fujian province died of a severe respiratory disease. Though she was buried before she could be examined, the girl's father and brother developed a similar illness, and tests confirmed both had an H5N1 virus. All the victims had visited relatives close to a region being hit by an unidentified virus.

The H5N1 that infected the family—and for that matter the birds—was not the same as the virus that hit Hong Kong in 1997. The original H5N1, and its many descendents and cousins, had spent the last five years mutating into thousands of related but new forms. For instance, the HA protein in the virus that killed the little girl came from the Hong Kong/1997 strain, but the NA protein and some other genes did not.

China's government, however, insisted it didn't have an avian influenza problem.

In 2003, H5N1 swept out of southern China and infected domesticated birds in Thailand. Poultry farming is one of Thailand's important business sectors. Poultry producers have enormous influence on the government, and on the mostly poor farmers who rely on them to buy birds. Though aware influenza had crossed the border, the government, at the request of big business, discouraged the farmers and scientists from speaking out. At the same time, poultry corporations cut prices to record lows to sell tons of potentially diseased meat in foreign countries.

In mid-January of 2004, Thailand's prime minister ate chicken on TV to dismiss the bird flu reports. But it became harder to hide the outbreak. On January 23, the government owned up to widespread bird flu in the northern provinces and more scattered outbreaks in the south. As the cover-up

Thailand's prime minister, Thaksin Shinawatra, publicly eating chicken in 2004 to dismiss bird flu reports in the country. *(Courtesy of AP Images)*

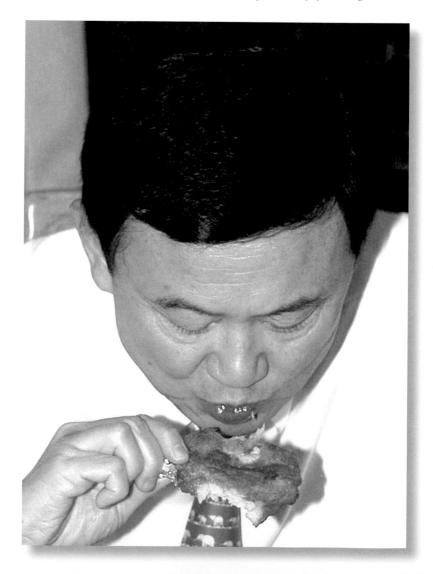

came to light, the World Health Organization and other public health organizations were aghast. Scandal roiled Thai politics. Meanwhile, several countries banned imports of chicken from the country.

From then on, bird flu turned up across East Asia. Before the end of January, Japan, Cambodia, South Korea, and Laos had confirmed cases in poultry. Indonesia reported H5N1 on February 2. By August it surfaced in Malaysia. Avian influenza had never spread so far, so fast.

Human cases, meanwhile, showed up in Vietnam and Thailand. The Vietnamese outbreak killed four out of four victims in July and August. In 2004-2005, a total of thirty-eight people died.

In early 2005, H5N1 claimed five people in Cambodia. By the end of the year, Indonesia had twenty cases. Reports of sick people continued to come in from Thailand and China.

A disturbing case occurred in Thailand. Investigators there found a sick girl had passed H5N1 to her mother, a woman named Pranee Thonghan. The person-to-person transmission, while troubling, did come with extenuating circumstances. Thonghan had closely tended her dying child, exposing herself to bodily fluids as well as the girl's coughing and breathing. But at the time, it looked like another near miss with a pandemic virus.

H5N1, in the meantime, expanded its range beyond *Homo sapiens*.

Cats, as far as anyone knew, didn't catch influenza of any kind. Then, in Thailand, a pair of tigers and a pair of panthers caught H5N1 from infected chicken carcasses. This was a prelude to a devastating outbreak at another Thai zoo in October 2004. Infected chicken meat again started the

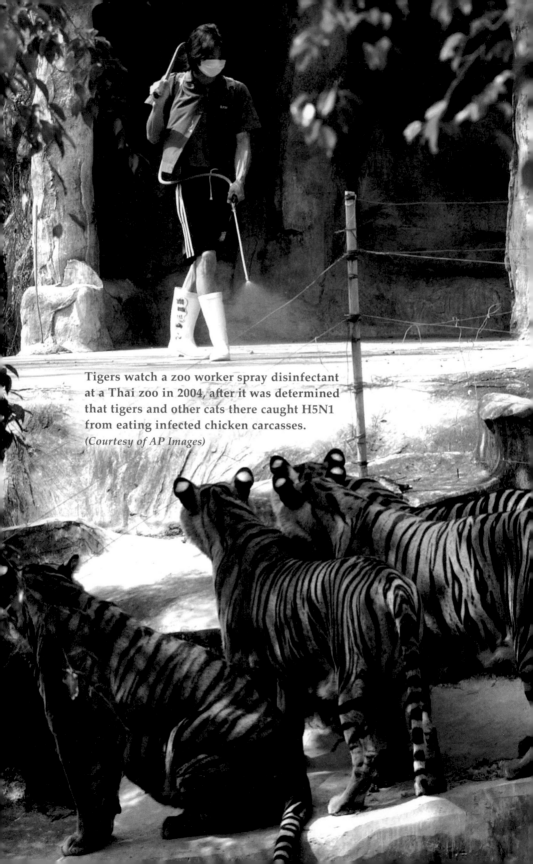

Tigers watch a zoo worker spray disinfectant at a Thai zoo in 2004, after it was determined that tigers and other cats there caught H5N1 from eating infected chicken carcasses. *(Courtesy of AP Images)*

trouble. This time, 147 tigers died or had to be put down. As research showed, cats not only caught H5N1, they spread it to other cats.

Lethal new forms of H5N1 had also begun to infect, and kill, wild birds. Until 2004, scientists thought wild birds didn't die of H5N1 viruses, or other kinds of flu, for that matter.

That H5N1 had changed became clear in the spring of 2005. A huge outbreak hit birds at Qinghai Lake, in China. Authorities counted 6,345 dead birds belonging to dozens of species, including migrating waterfowl. The culprit turned out to be a previously unknown kind of H5N1. In lab tests, it ruthlessly killed birds and mice.

Scientists began to look for evidence that geese, mallard ducks (the most efficient spreader), and other migratory species might be dropping avian flu virus along their migratory routes. Reports of bird die-offs came in from Siberia, from Kazakhstan, from Mongolia.

It wasn't just the wild birds, though. Influenza burned through Asia's domesticated poultry flocks. Disease and slaughters to prevent it from spreading killed 100 million chickens in a matter of months. Despite the culls, however, bird flu returned in 2005, 2006, and 2007.

"The evidence is now overwhelming that migrating birds can move H5N1 over long distances," said Malik Peiris, a flu expert at the University of Hong Kong. "But they are not scapegoats for maintaining H5N1 within poultry. There the cause and solution lies within the poultry industry."

H5N1 viruses had found a niche in both domesticated and wild birds. That being the case, experts admitted there was no

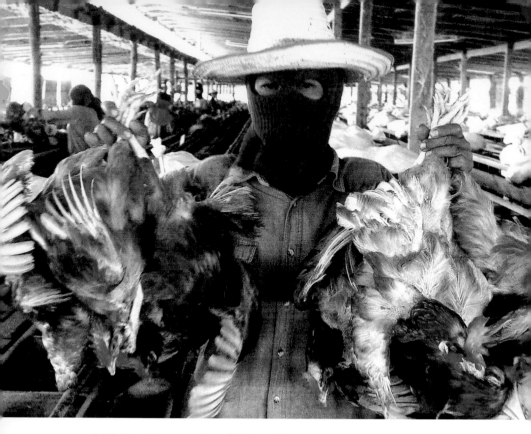
A Thai worker carrying chickens during a chicken purge in 2004.
(*Courtesy of AP Images*)

way to stop its spread. A new scenario came into play. Wild birds carried the virus to new places. Once there, domesticated birds caught it and, through force of numbers, amplified it into a threat.

H5N1 arrived in Europe by October 2005. Romania reported cases in domestic poultry, and Croatia in dead wild swans. One month later, an H5N1-infected flamingo turned up in Kuwait, the Middle East's first case. Nigeria, the first African country to report, found H5N1 in domesticated poultry in February 2006. An outbreak hit a British poultry farm eleven months later.

The number of human cases was also on the rise. In autumn 2005, avian influenza hit the Turkish poultry indus-

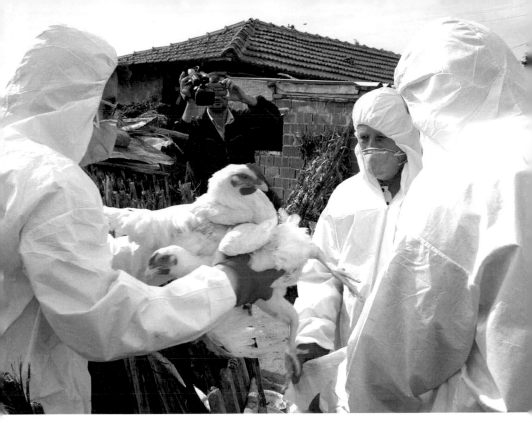

Officials collecting chickens to fight a flu outbreak in western Turkey in 2005. *(Courtesy of AP Images)*

try, leading the European Union to ban certain products. Early the following year, six people in and near the village of Dogubayazit caught H5N1. Four of them, all children, had reportedly been playing with the head of a dead chicken. New cases soon appeared around Ankara, the Turkish capital. The Turkish government launched a mass slaughter.

The Turkish outbreak totaled twelve confirmed human cases, with four deaths. The virus was genetically close to the H5N1 found in dead birds at Qinghai Lake. Genetic tests on viruses found in Nigeria also showed a similar relationship. This suggested—some experts said it confirmed—that the viruses rode along with migratory birds.

At the end of 2006, renewed human outbreaks shook Indonesia and Egypt.

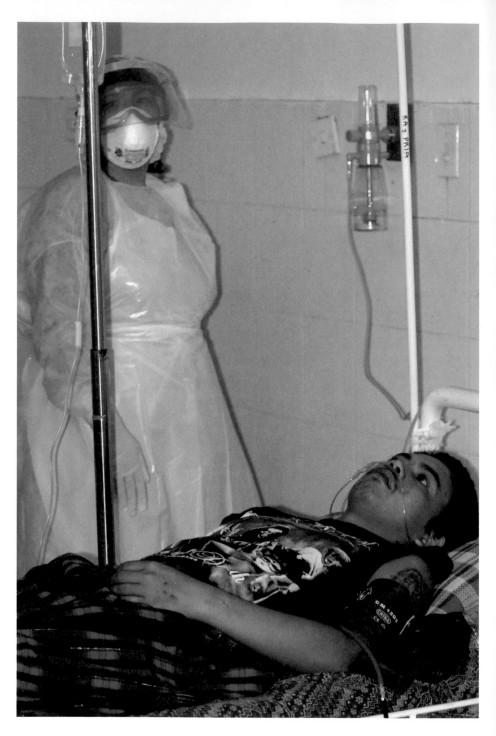

A bird flu victim at an Indonesian hospital in 2006. *(Courtesy of AP Images)*

Since H5N1's arrival in 2004, Indonesia had become one of the countries hardest hit by the disease. The first human case was reported in July 2005. Over the next seven months, Indonesia discovered twenty-five total cases. Eighteen of the victims died. The number of cases doubled by the summer of 2006. By the following January, the count had reached eighty-one, the second most behind Vietnam.

Antigenic drift continued throughout the period. Not every one of the viruses posed a danger. Milder H5N1s were also winging to new countries with wild waterfowl.

One mutant virus stood out, however. Starting at the beginning of 2002, viruses belonging to the "Z" group dominated in southern China. One of the viruses, called Z+, was behind the spread of avian flu through Southeast Asia in 2003, and, especially, in 2004. Z+ was lethal. It spread efficiently. It evolved fast and continued to trade genes with other flu viruses as it traveled across regions and jumped from species to species.

Mice, usually immune to influenza, caught and always died from Z+. It took only a miniscule amount to pass it to them. Chicken embryos infected with it died in a couple of days—an obstacle to both research and producing vaccines.

Like so much influenza, Z+ was hard to predict. By constantly infecting chickens, it mutated into a form more lethal to them, and, as events in Asia showed, killed them by the thousands. Yet the same virus infected domesticated ducks *without* harming them.

And H5N1's mutation continues. In a year's time, a formerly minor strain known as Fujian-like (after Fujian, a region in China) increased its spread until, in February 2007, it caused the vast majority of southern China's known avian flu infections. (The Chinese government denied the Fujian-like

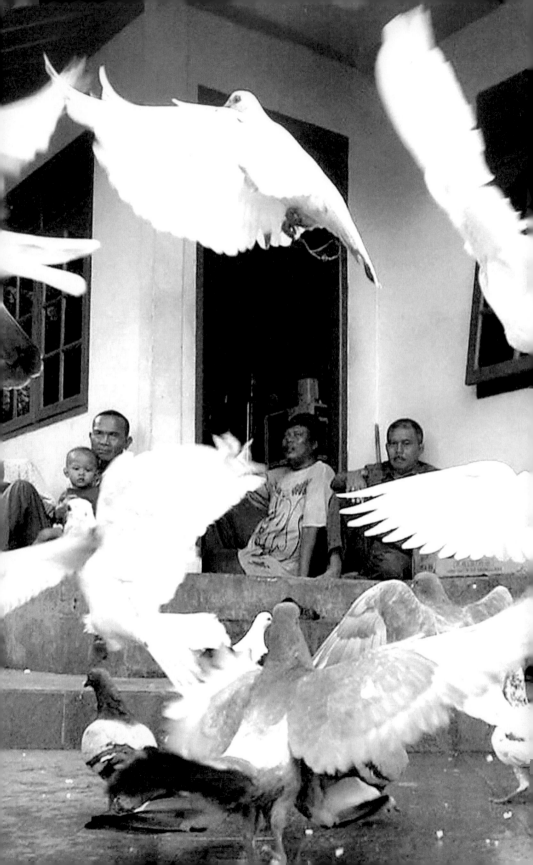

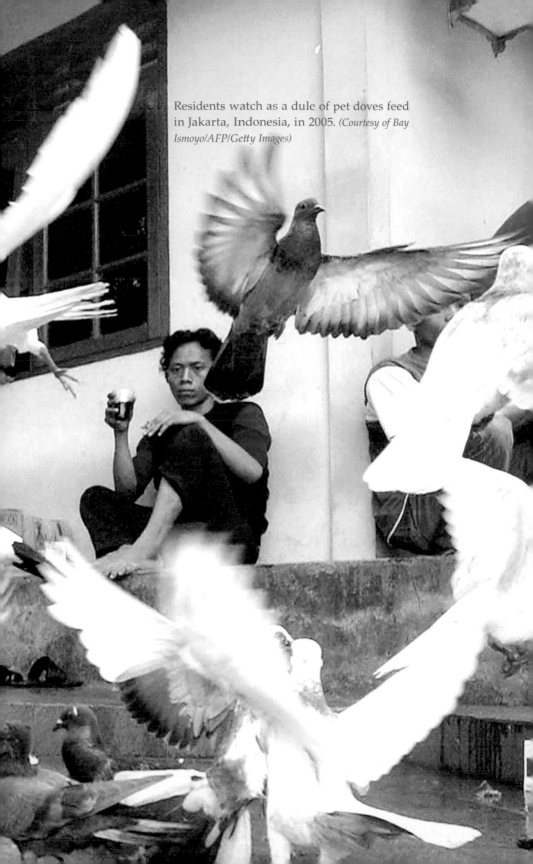

Residents watch as a dule of pet doves feed in Jakarta, Indonesia, in 2005. *(Courtesy of Bay Ismoyo/AFP/Getty Images)*

virus existed.) It spread to neighboring Thailand and Laos, and farther south to Malaysia. Experts fear a strain as dominant as Fujian-like could set off another explosive round of epidemics in birds throughout Asia.

While scientists waited to see what the Fujian-like virus would do next, H5N1 continued to infect humans. Indonesia counted nineteen deaths in the first five months of 2007, bringing the total to seventy-seven. By May of 2007, H5N1 avian influenza had killed human beings in twelve countries. It still raged among domesticated birds in Egypt, Indonesia, and Nigeria, had forced Ghana to cull poultry, and turned up in Pakistan. China, secretive as always, refused to own up to what the disease was doing inside its borders. Where H5N1 would appear next, and the form it would take, remained uncertain.

The Hunt for the Spanish Flu

In 1995, a scientist at the Armed Forces Institute of Pathology (AFIP) named Jeffrey Taubenberger was looking to tackle a historical mystery. The AFIP was founded in 1862 as the Army Medical Museum, with a focus on searching for ways to fight battlefield diseases. Toward that end, it collected and archived tissue of all kinds from solders, sailors, marines, and other members of the armed services. In almost a century prior to 1995, the AFIP's archive—the National Tissue Repository—had acquired more than two-and-a-half million samples.

Taubenberger specialized in finding genetic material from these kinds of old tissue, preserved as they are on slides or under wax or in jars filled with Formaldehyde, a preservative. Working with Ann Reid, a technician, Taubenberger set out to see if the Spanish flu virus had survived in one or more of the warehoused tissue samples.

In the summer of 1996, the AFIP team focused on the case of a soldier named Roscoe Vaughan. Vaughan, aged twenty-one, had reported sick on September 19 at Fort Jackson, South Carolina. A week later he died, one of his lungs destroyed by aggressive pneumonia. Doctors took a tissue sample during the autopsy. Following the usual procedure, they put the sample in Formaldehyde, covered it in paraffin, and sent it to the archive.

Taubenberger's team, using advanced microbiological techniques, recovered genetic fragments of the Spanish flu virus from Vaughan's sample, proving that scientists could dig out influenza's genetic material from old tissue. Once published, the findings became a national news story, with the AFIP team hailed as the discoverers of the long-lost Spanish flu.

But science is about confirmation. To prove Vaughan really died of Spanish flu, Taubenberger and his team needed to compare the virus they had found to that from another victim.

Johan Hultin was a retired pathologist born in Sweden and living in northern California. Seeing Taubenberger's article in *Science*, Hultin wrote him a letter explaining his own extraordinary background with the Spanish flu virus.

In 1951, while in graduate school, Hultin had flown to Alaska as part of a team to investigate the mass graves of Native Americans killed by the disease. The group hoped samples of the virus could be taken from victims buried in permafrost. Though Hultin obtained tissue samples, he failed to isolate the virus in the laboratory.

In his letter, Hultin volunteered to pay his own way back to Alaska to try again. Taubenberger accepted the offer. Once in Teller Mission (now renamed Brevig Mission), Hultin asked permission to exhume 1918 flu victims. Village leaders agreed.

Hultin, assisted by four local men, describes finding the corpse of a young woman named Lucy.

> I sat on a pail—turned upside down—and looked at her. Then I saw it. She was an obese woman; she had fat in her skin and around her organs and that served as a protection from the occasional short-term thawing of permafrost. Those on either side of her were not obese and they had decayed. I . . . saw this woman in a state of good preservation. And I knew this was where the virus has got to come from.

Hultin cut out Lucy's lungs and, along with samples from three other corpses, stored the organs and tissue in preservatives. Soon after, he divided the material into four packages and sent them to Taubenberger.

Over the next three weeks, Taubenberger recovered fragments of Spanish flu RNA from the lungs taken out of Lucy. His team matched the RNA that Hultin had found, plus that of another dead WWI soldier they had obtained, against Vaughn, the original case. The three viruses had only minor differences. Vaughn, indeed, had Spanish flu.

Over the next eight years, Taubenberger led the effort to learn the virus's entire genetic structure. At each step he and his team published more of the sequence, a decision that caused controversy in the scientific community. The September 11, 2001, terrorist attacks and the still-unsolved anthrax mailings that followed brought up worries about biological terrorism—and how a terrorist group might use the genetic sequences to recreate, and then release, Spanish flu.

Work nonetheless went ahead. The October 6, 2005, issue of the journal *Nature* published the codes of the last three genes. From that moment, Spanish flu's entire genetic structure was available to the public.

The same week, the Centers for Disease Control announced a breakthrough of its own. A team led by Terence Tumpey, senior microbiologist at the CDC's Influenza Branch, announced it had used Taubenberger's work to make a living copy of the Spanish flu virus.

A number of important findings came out of both teams' research. In 2005, they discovered the 1918 virus

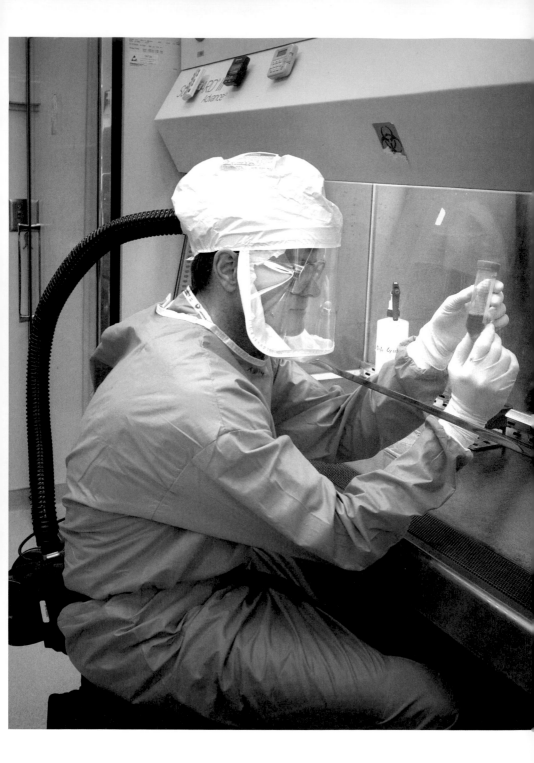

Dr. Terrence Tumpey examining a reconstructed 1918 Spanish flu virus.
(Courtesy of Centers for Disease Control and Prevention)

crawled deeper into the lungs than a usual influenza strain, down into the alveoli where oxygen and carbon dioxide were exchanged. Also, the virus turned out to be an avian influenza, rather than a reassortant of a human and bird flu.

Tumpey's work, and that of others, continues to explore what made the 1918 virus tick.

Despite the flood of new information, concerns about terrorism revived after the publication of the Spanish flu genome. One bacteriologist called it "the most effective bioweapons agent now known."

Tumpey responded that the chance to learn canceled out the risks. "For the first time we have a truly avian pandemic influenza virus that we can study," he said. That could help researchers learn what combination of genetic factors led to killer pandemic strains. Those factors, once known, could be watched for as new viruses evolved and appeared.

seven
Surveillance and Preparation

Influenza experts disagree on many things, but there's one point that inspires agreement: there will be another influenza pandemic. It's just a question of when. And as with many kinds of natural disasters, *When?* is a question scientists can't answer for certain.

What? poses the same problem. We don't yet know what this pandemic virus can do, for the simple reason it has yet to evolve into existence. Whether it will be mild or severe, whether it will prefer young victims or the old, what it will do to the body—all are unknowable.

But major public health institutions like the Centers for Disease Control and the World Health Organization have made predictions. A repeat of a relatively mild pandemic virus like the 1968 Hong Kong flu would kill at least 89,000 Americans, according to the CDC. The death toll could run as high as 207,000.

A Spanish flu-like pandemic would be far worse. If just a quarter of the American population caught such a virus, about 75 million people would get sick. An estimated two to two-and-a-half percent of those infected with Spanish flu died. A virus with the same fatality rate would kill approximately 1.8 million Americans. If a new pandemic virus killed at the rate the H5N1s do in Asia, the toll might soar to 14 million, with a huge percentage of victims under age thirty-five.

Poorer countries would suffer more. Health systems there lack the antibiotics, respirators, advanced laboratories, and trained medical professionals that in the wealthy countries would save some lives.

Poverty would also intensify a pandemic flu's effects in other ways. Conditions in refugee camps and the shantytowns that ring cities in the developing world encourage disease. As many as 200,000 people may pack into a typical square mile of space. They live without health care, and face primitive

A view of slums in São Paulo, Brazil. Conditions in shantytowns such as this encourage the development and spread of sicknesses like the flu.

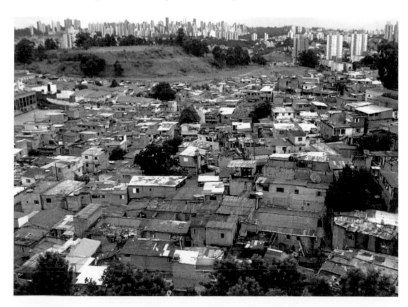

sewage systems, poor air quality, rampant garbage, abundant animal pests, and other problems that put pressure on their health.

Poverty can also bring people into increased contact with influenza. Poor Nigerians, seeking a cheap meal, have bought flu-ridden birds at a discount—and taken dead chickens from city dumps.

Air travel would also spread influenza faster than was possible in 1918. Hong Kong, for example, is a transportation hub used by thousands of travelers every day. Flights leave the city around the clock. A single sick passenger might infect dozens of people over the course of a flight. By the time any of them showed symptoms, they'd be scattered to their homes or businesses, to vacation spots, or on connecting flights elsewhere.

Planes at an airport in Hong Kong. The frequency of air travel today would spread influenza faster than was possible in 1918.

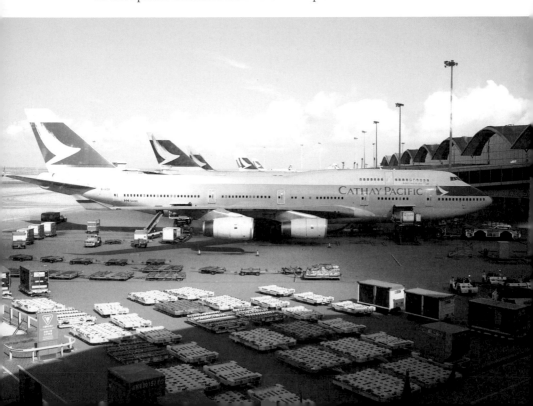

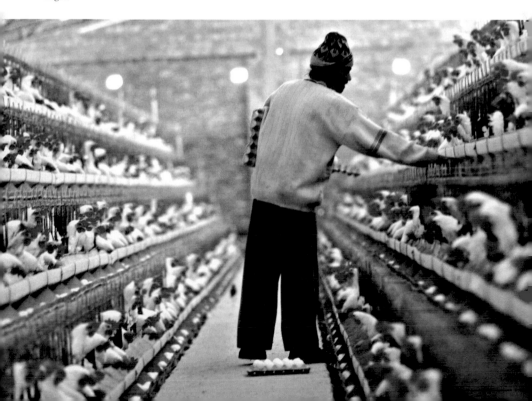

Another aspect of the contemporary world, the way we raise livestock, encourages the virus to evolve in new directions.

Since 1980, the worldwide consumption of meat has skyrocketed. The biggest part of the increase has occurred in the parts of the developing world where economic progress has given consumers enough money to add meat, especially pork and chicken, to their diet. Because of the increased demand, family farms are giving way to an industrialized system that breeds, raises, and slaughters livestock on a mass scale.

Factory farms sit at the hub of the system. Today's facilities are overcrowded pig and chicken cities where animals are raised in small spaces in close contact with others of

A laborer collecting eggs at a poultry farm in northern India. Farms like this, in which animals are kept in small spaces and in close contact with each other, encourages the spread and evolution of the flu virus. *(Courtesy of AP Images)*

their kind. The numbers are astonishing. In places like western Arkansas and northern Georgia, the American poultry industry may kill a billion birds per year and can crank out 20 million pounds of chicken meat every day.

Some facilities pack 50,000 birds into a two-story building. A single factory farm complex might hold up to a million birds.

Swine farming has experienced a similar change. The world pig population has already topped 1 billion, a number unprecedented in history. Some observers believe the number will double by the year 2020 to keep up with increasing demand.

An animal city, like a human one, produces mountains of waste. When it comes to influenza, that's a problem, because a chicken excretes virus. Birds living under factory farm conditions have contact with one-another's waste, breath, blood, and mucus, as well as food and drinking water. An egg infected with virus can spread it to chicks in an incubator. Employees can track it from building to building, or from one region to another, on their boots.

The constant swapping of influenza viruses between sick birds accelerates avian flu's already dynamic mutation rate. Even vaccines used to protect livestock can encourage antigenic drift. Selection pressure, again, comes into play. Animal flu vaccines are widely used, and necessary, to protect against recognized flu viruses. Those well-known strains, unable to find victims in a vaccinated flock, disappear. In Darwinist terms, they can no longer compete. Vaccines basically push a virus to mutate or perish.

An unfamiliar strain, however, continues to reproduce—to out-compete—the others, because vaccines don't stop it.

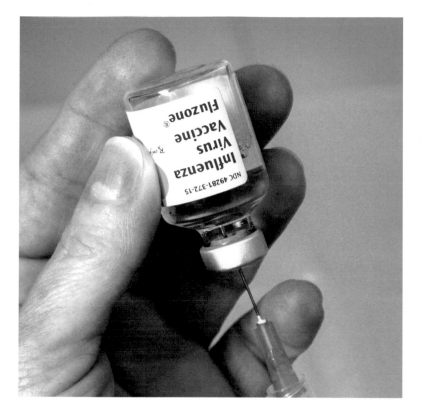

Influenza virus vaccine being extracted from a vial. While getting vaccinated is an important part of flu prevention, researchers have yet to create a vaccine that protects against all influenza viruses. *(Courtesy of Centers for Disease Control and Prevention)*

This virus takes over and starts infecting the birds or pigs. If created in time, a vaccine can be made to stop it too. If not, the mutant virus spreads in secret. On rare occasions, this new kind of influenza gets loose and causes an explosive outbreak.

One of the worst of these rare outbreaks took place in 2003, in the Netherlands. The country leads the world in the export of eggs and live chickens, and has a thriving industry in other kinds of poultry. In addition, wild migratory birds share the country's famous canals and wetlands with domestic birds kept on family farms. Both situations offer influenza an opportunity. An outbreak of an avian virus—classified as an H7N7, not the better-known H5N1—forced the Dutch to slaughter 30 million chickens. When the virus appeared in pigs, the government culled the entire swine population.

Animals weren't the only ones affected. Nine workers involved in the slaughter developed mild flu symptoms. Far more people, 2,000 out of 4,500, picked up the infection without knowing it. Some in turn passed the virus on to others. Though the symptoms were almost always mild (only one person, a veterinarian, died), the H7N7 definitely passed person-to-person.

The Netherlands outbreak showed viruses that incubated on farms could get into human populations. Transportation adds to the risks. In the U.S., for example, both swine and poultry are trucked all over the country. The animals can spread a virus to new regions or, as happened in 2002 in California, to farms they pass on the way.

Even during outbreaks, when governments may ban the transport of birds, smugglers help viruses spread. An estimated ten tons of smuggled chicken crosses from China to Vietnam every day. Inspecting each shipment across long borders, especially the leaky borders common in developing countries, is impossible.

A bird slaughter, while necessary at times, has its own hazards. Sweeping up and disinfecting bird corpses bring workers closer to the virus. So does heaping dead chickens into piles for burning, or throwing dead turkeys into trenches to be buried. Providing protective gear costs more than many

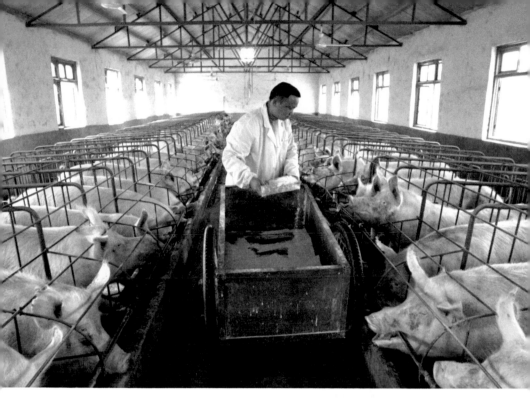

A Chinese farmer feeding pigs at a pig farm in 2007. The current increasing demand for meat leads to large factory farms that increase the opportunity for animal and human diseases to spread. (*Courtesy of AP Images*)

governments can, or will, pay. And, as in the Netherlands, doing so may not prevent infection anyway.

These factors led one study to conclude that the livestock revolution of the past few decades has increased the odds of unleashing infectious pathogens. And influenza isn't the only one, by any means. Changes in the way livestock is fed have exposed humans to bovine spongiform encephalopathy ("mad cow disease").

These increased dangers seem more ominous when you realize China, long considered a source of influenza pandemics, has embraced industrial farming on an immense scale.

In 1983, China produced 16 million metric tons of meat. By 2020 demand for pork and poultry is expected to put that figure closer to 107 million metric tons. The United Nations lists China as the world's biggest producer of chicken, duck, and goose eaten by human beings.

Rising demand means more and bigger factory farms with chickens, pigs, and humans in contact with each other—and each other's influenza because, while China's poultry industry approaches that in America for hugeness, the standards for cleanliness and disease prevention are far lower.

Both ducks and chickens are farmed in huge numbers. One source puts the chicken population in Guangdong province at 700 million birds. Wild species and domesticated ones have a lot of contact because of declining wetlands and wild birds' love of poaching a free meal from farms.

The region's role in the global economy makes it important beyond influenza. Cell phones, computer components, toys, athletic shoes—Guangdong manufactures these products and a lot more for sale around the world. In the event of a pandemic, Guangdong factories might not be able to fill orders for exports like computer chips. Any interruption in deliveries would affect high-tech industry on every continent.

The same goes for other goods. According to Dr. Michael Osterholm of the University of Minnesota's Center for Infectious Disease, "Under a moderate to severe pandemic, developed-world countries that rely on a constant supply of pharmaceutical and medical products would see an interruption in trade and travel. Essential products like that will not be available."

When a pandemic strain does appear, public health officials and scientists hope to stamp it out before it spreads too far.

To that end, international agencies like the WHO have initiated new surveillance programs and expanded old ones. A web of 122 facilities in ninety-four countries tracks influenza to see what it is and how it's mutating. A number of other laboratories occasionally send in viruses that they have found too. National Influenza Centers gather approximately 175,000 samples per year of various flu viruses.

WHO Collaborating Centers in London, Tokyo, Melbourne, and at the CDC in Atlanta form the backbone of the surveillance network. These four institutions analyze (at no cost) a fraction of the virus samples to determine their genetic structure. The Collaborating Centers also offer advice and provide other services.

Individual nations have also begun their own surveillance programs. In 2006, the U.S. government began to watch migrating birds—and especially ducks, geese, and shorebirds—to see if the animals have carried in H5N1 viruses from Asia. Investigators test live wild birds and those killed by hunters, as well as disease-free birds relocated to wetlands. Water and bird feces are also sampled. The collected information goes into a database for use by various government agencies and scientific institutions.

Though testing takes place nationwide, the program pays special attention to Alaska and the Pacific coast—places where Asian species mingle with North American birds.

By watching birds, scientists hope to stop a dangerous bird flu virus from gaining a foothold in North America. "The best defense against emerging and epidemic-prone diseases is not passive barriers at borders, airports, and seaports," said Margaret Chan, director-general of the WHO. "It is proactive risk management that seeks to detect an outbreak early and stop it at its source—before it has a chance to become an international threat."

In addition to national programs, experts have drawn up a list of suggested preventative measures for use around the world. The suggestions include:

* Teaching Asia's small-scale farmers, and others who keep poultry, how to raise and slaughter birds without exposing themselves to risk

* Separating swine and poultry

* Keeping domesticated flocks away from wild birds, with special attention paid to places visited by migrating waterfowl and sea birds

* The use of chlorine or other methods to treat water used by at-risk wild birds to kill any virus

* Vaccination of poultry

* Disinfecting and washing any vehicle or equipment that leaves a poultry farm

* Avoiding other farms and markets where birds are kept, or wearing different boots and clothes if doing so is necessary

* Reporting all suspected cases of avian flu

Though the measures sound basic, it's hard to get people to comply. The biggest problem is money. Countries wanting to participate often lack the resources to fund surveillance and vaccination programs. But other issues arise.

Governments cover up outbreaks for economic reasons. Nations might ban imports from infected countries, at the cost of billions of dollars. It happened in 1994 in India, when a number of countries boycotted Indian products because of a pneumonic plague outbreak.

Corporations have the same incentive. Or a company may choose to save money with inadequate protective gear or by ignoring regulations.

Small-scale farmers play an essential role in surveillance because they are on the front lines, working with birds every day. Yet they sometimes don't report avian flu, afraid they'll lose their birds—and their investment in the birds—to a government-ordered cull.

To encourage better surveillance, Indonesia's government promised to pay for each slaughtered bird. The country's flu risk is high. According to Indonesia's chief veterinarian, 80 percent of Indonesians raise poultry, either on farms or in their backyards. But the government's voucher system didn't

Workers throw bags containing dead chickens into a dump site in 2004. Chicken farmers are often hesitant to report cases of bird flu, out of fear their animals will all be taken away and slaughtered. *(Courtesy of AP Images)*

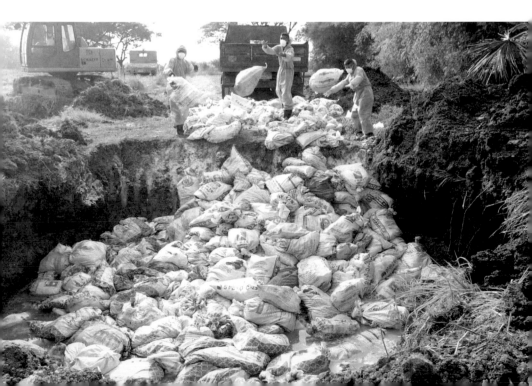

inspire confidence. Indonesians, shrugging off dead chickens and what they see as a handful of human deaths, went on raising birds and reporting or not reporting influenza, as they saw fit.

At the same time, the high costs of compensating farmers makes Chinese officials reluctant to order culls or even report outbreaks. Some farmers in Laos reportedly ate their chickens rather than turn them over for slaughter.

With so much at stake, it's easy to forget that, from the farmers' point of view, avian influenza isn't a national or international problem. It's a personal one that threatens their well-being. "Pay attention to us, too, the little people who earn our living as poultry traders," one Indonesian poultry trader said. "Don't wipe out the disease by destroying all the chickens. . . . If this happens, how will we earn our living? Our children need money to go to school."

Then there's politics. When H5N1 first appeared in Vietnam, the government made a show of "proving" it could handle the situation without aid from the international community. But its vaccination program failed, and its announced cures didn't line up with scientific facts.

Political rivalries also cross over into the scientific community. By late 2006, Indonesia had recorded one hundred eight deaths from avian influenza, the most in the world. But the country's government ceased sharing virus samples with the WHO in protest over drug companies using the samples to make (and profit from) vaccines that Indonesians were too poor to buy.

Without samples from Indonesia, the world community cannot track H5N1. That kind of hole in the international surveillance system could allow the virus to mutate into a pandemic

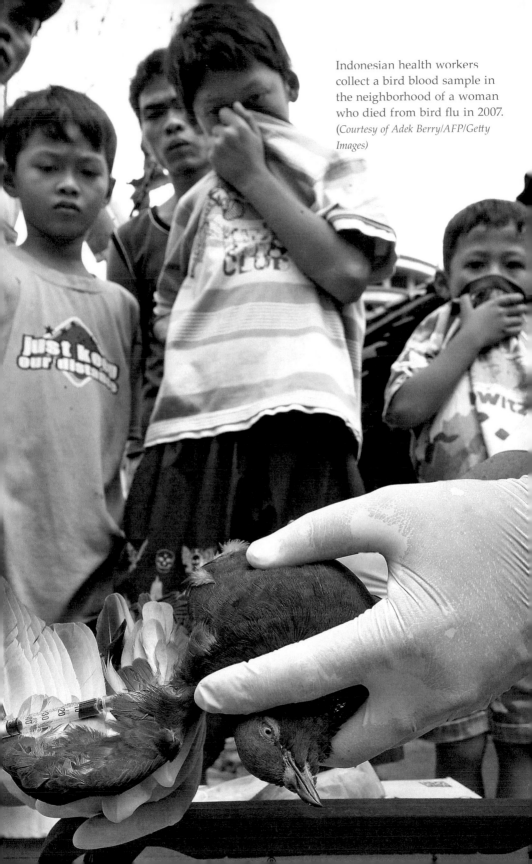

Indonesian health workers collect a bird blood sample in the neighborhood of a woman who died from bird flu in 2007. *(Courtesy of Adek Berry/AFP/Getty Images)*

form and get loose before anyone realizes it has changed. As it stands, it would take at least six months to get a vaccine to the public. Indonesia's unwillingness to share samples could delay that timetable.

China and Vietnam also have withheld essential material like throat cultures and blood samples. But richer countries come in for criticism too. Scientists at research institutions sometimes keep data and findings until they publish it. Publishing research in scientific journals plays a major part in a person's career, helping to find better jobs and win grant money.

Indonesia took things a step further in mid-2008 by stating it would no longer tell global health organizations about individual avian influenza cases and instead would announce totals every six months. The country's health minister, Siti Fadilah Supari, cited negative reactions by the media and outside experts as reason for the policy change. Critics have responded by stating that a lack of surveillance in the country hardest hit by avian influenza might allow a pandemic-capable H5N1 to appear and take hold before global health organizations could stop it.

Negotiations have made progress on the various issues, albeit only a little at a time. In 2006, China, after dragging its feet for more than two years, agreed to provide H5N1 samples from the Qinghai Lake. Samples from human avian flu cases were also sent. Scientists praised the move as a breakthrough.

Of all the obstacles to effective surveillance, lack of money may be the hardest to overcome. The big international agencies like the WHO can devote only a small percentage of its budget to flu-related activities. With that money the WHO must maintain its laboratory system, investigate outbreaks, lobby governments to both improve public health and be honest about influenza, and negotiate problems in areas like vaccine manufacturing.

The UN's Food and Agricultural Organization, with similar funding problems, leads the effort to monitor animal populations. But with H5N1 spreading, the area that needs to be watched keeps getting bigger.

Poor countries have even less chance of coping. As avian influenza emerged across Southeast Asia, a lack of money, equipment, and facilities hampered the effort to control it. In Vietnam, the nation's main laboratory went into an investigation without masks or gloves.

Furthermore, influenza is just one of a long list of issues these governments have to address. All the countries have millions of citizens living in poverty. All deal with serious public health problems: high infant mortality, a surge in exotic diseases like dengue fever, a range of gastrointestinal and respiratory problems. Many face natural disasters too, whether monsoon floods in Bangladesh or volcanoes in Indonesia.

The flip side of surveillance is planning what to do if an influenza pandemic occurs.

Undoubtedly, most of the world would have to rely on wealthy nations—the U.S., Canada, western Europe, Japan, Australia—to supply expertise, vaccines and medicine, money, and an example of how to cope. If those nations were swamped by the pandemic, the effects in poorer countries left on their own might be unthinkable.

National governments, responsible for their own citizens, play the vital role in pandemic preparedness. In the U.S., the federal government and many local governments have drawn up plans. Guidelines released in February of 2007 suggest the sick and anyone in contact with them, healthy or otherwise, remain isolated at home for a week to ten days. Local governments were asked to provide for the elderly, the handicapped, and other groups who'd face special difficulties.

The Spanish flu pandemic influenced many of the other suggestions. For instance, in a severe pandemic, communities should close public places like schools, day-care centers,

U.S. Health and Human Services Secretary Michael Leavitt addresses a 2006 gathering of public health officials to discuss ways to prepare for a possible bird flu outbreak. *(Courtesy of AP Images)*

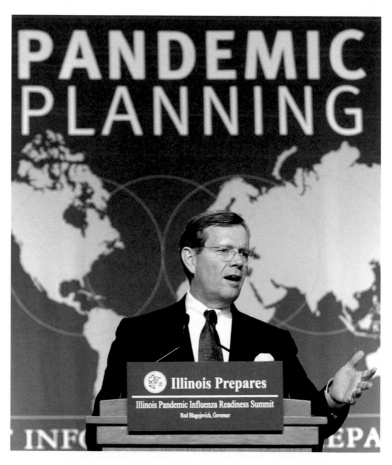

and churches, cancel or curb public transportation, ask people to avoid crowds, provide antiviral drugs, and start face mask programs. Not every expert agrees with the entire list—masks may not prevent transmission of the virus, for one thing—but it's a start.

As one researcher put it, the guidelines won't stop influenza from spreading, but they might cut the number of cases and, therefore, the number of deaths. Computer models running data from the 1918 pandemic suggest that such measures, if put in place in time and maintained until the pandemic passes, may have kept down the death rate.

Delaying the spread also might give scientists and drug manufacturers time to find, and produce, an effective vaccine.

Some states have used drills to test their response systems. A vaccination exercise in two Washington state counties showed officials they needed to print written matter in more languages and to plan for bad weather. These kinds of "war games" help governments work out potential problems before, not after, a pandemic arrives.

Experts praise the plans but point to holes. Some countries, for instance, have stockpiled Tamiflu, the major anti-influenza medicine. Tamiflu (generic name oseltamivir) works by blocking the work done by the neuraminidase protein. This keeps influenza virus from escaping an infected cell; the copies of virus, stuck, die there without a chance to infect new cells. Tamiflu doesn't prevent influenza, however. It merely holds down the virus and shortens the length of the illness. Victims can remain contagious.

Tamiflu has other limits. A victim must start taking the tablets within thirty-six hours of exposure to a virus. With

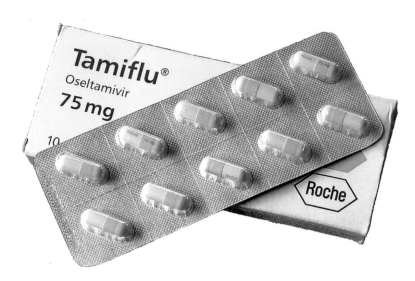

Although Tamiflu is expensive and its effectiveness is limited, it is viewed as an important antiflu drug.

some people, it takes that long (or longer) for symptoms to appear, and when it happens, there's no guarantee a victim will know it's influenza. By the time they go to the doctor, the window to best use the drug may have closed.

Nor is Tamiflu cheap. It costs about seventy dollars and up for a five-day course. (Governments buy it in bulk at a discount—fifteen dollars for poor countries, eighteen dollars for the rich ones.) Some scientists have also speculated that it may take twice as much Tamiflu, taken for seven to ten days, to knock down a severe pandemic-level virus.

To make matters worse, there are reports from Egypt that the strain of H5N1 in that country resists Tamiflu's effects.

The start of the 2008-2009 flu season brought the news that one of the major strains of human flu in circulation was also Tamiflu-resistant. Scientists had known for some time that many of the H1N1 viruses infecting human beings had begun to resist the drug. By 2007-2008, in fact, resistance was being seen across Europe, and forty countries reported resistant H1N1 during the first eight months of 2008. As a new Northern Hemisphere flu season got going at the end of 2008, early testing from the CDC suggested Tamiflu failed against a breathtaking 98 percent of the H1N1 strains submitted to the institution.

The majority opinion in the scientific community blamed a spontaneous genetic mutation. News stories, meanwhile, quoted experts surprised by the turn of events. "It's quite shocking," said Kent A. Sepkowitz of New York's Memorial Sloan-Kettering Cancer Center. "We've never lost an antimicrobial this fast. It blew me away." Yuan-Po Tu, an associate medical director at the Everett Clinic in Washington state, said, "We could lose a very, very useful drug very, very quickly."

As for the stockpiling strategy, no country has enough of the drug for all its citizens. Many haven't tried. Poor countries have little if any Tamiflu in stock.

If a pandemic struck the U.S. from coast to coast, supplies would run out fast. Buying more has become a problem too. Tamiflu's manufacturer cut back production in April 2007 due to lack of demand. Yet public health institutions from the WHO down will depend on the drug in case of a pandemic.

The other antiflu drugs present even more problems. Tamiflu's major competitor, Relenza (generic name zanamivir), acts in a similar way, but requires an inhaler, making it harder to use.

The WHO, nonetheless, suggested creating a sort of Tamiflu savings account. When pandemic influenza emerged, the drug would be rushed to the region to smother the virus with a "Tamiflu blanket" before it spread. Experience has showed the limits of the plan, however. Vietnam's army had taken the Tamiflu sent there in 2004. There was no reason to believe similar things wouldn't happen elsewhere.

There's also the question of how to handle the surge of sick people. In the past thirty years, American health care has, like the poultry industry, become enormous and focused on the bottom line. Experts, looking at years of budget cuts, worry the system isn't capable of handling the increased number of patients created by a pandemic, and sounded alarms about a lack of surge capacity—the ability of institutions to accommodate a spike in the number of sick people needing care.

The number of available beds in a hospital, especially an urban hospital, runs close to zero on an average day. A surge in influenza cases will quickly fill up the extra beds, and then some. Furthermore, other patients cannot be put on hold—people will still be giving birth and recovering from surgery. Just finding a place to put dozens or hundreds of infected (and contagious) flu victims will be a challenge.

Even if rooms could be found, streamlining has cut personnel, particularly when it comes to nurses and support staff like orderlies. As a result, there may not be enough caregivers to treat and clean up after the sick. On top of that, basic supplies—not just vaccine and Tamiflu but masks, food, needles, and linen—would run out fast unless stockpiled beforehand. That's not being done.

Our infrastructure in general faces the same problem. If millions are on their backs with flu, who drives the gasoline trucks? Delivers the food? Fights the fires? The world won't end, of course. But during the pandemic's peak, a period of a few weeks, society may be stretched to the limit. A power outage caused by a blizzard may last days rather than hours.

If it happened during January in a northern city, cold-related fatalities might drive the death toll higher. Certainly it would add to the misery and panic.

Despite the obstacles, however, there are reasons for hope.

Influenza is a familiar disease and, with so much talk of bird flu, physicians have a heightened awareness of it. Some argue that modern medicine, so much better now than in 1918, will be able to do far more to keep victims alive and to keep others from getting sick. (Not everyone agrees.)

Researchers are also learning more about the disease. If a pandemic doesn't show up first, it's possible we'll make major progress in finding influenza, preventing it, diagnosing it, and treating it. Perhaps we'll be able to prevent, or at least curb, a pandemic virus before a repeat of 1918 can take place.

More nations than ever take influenza surveillance seriously. While work remains to be done, negotiation and education have encouraged avian flu hot spots like Indonesia and Thailand to act more wisely and more decisively than even a few years ago. China, though still a concern, has pledged better cooperation, with providing lab samples at the top of the list.

It may be that the H5N1 missed its chance to become a pandemic. Some scientists think so. "For years they have been telling us it's going to happen—and it hasn't," said Jeremy Farrar, a physician at the Hospital for Tropical Disease in Ho Chi Minh City, Vietnam. "Billions of chickens in Asia have been infected and millions of people lived with them . . . and less than 200 people have gotten infected. . . . That tells you the constraints on the virus are considerable.

It must be hard for this virus to jump."

The virus, it turns out, may have bad aim. Ordinary human influenza favors cells that line the upper respiratory system—the nose and throat. Avian viruses, however, find it easiest to attack cells in the deepest part of the lungs. Once there, avian flu can be devastating. But its inability to find a grip in the nose and throat delays it from going any further.

When it comes to protecting against pandemic flu, experts and the public look to vaccines.

On the good side, the U.S. Food and Drug Administration approved a basic vaccine against H5N1 viruses in April 2007. The emergency-only vaccine generated immunity in about 45 percent of the people who got it, but each person needed two shots given a month apart, and it took twelve times as much vaccine as an ordinary flu shot. Still, it represents progress. Eventually, scientists hope to build on the existing H5N1 vaccine and create a more reliable version that could be given in smaller doses to protect people until a vaccine focused on the specific pandemic virus could be developed.

Researchers are also looking for a "universal vaccine" that protects against all influenza viruses. The universal vaccine is years away, though, assuming one is even possible.

The main obstacle to a vaccine against a pandemic is that we have no idea what the pandemic virus will look like. Since a vaccine requires a sample of the specific virus, work can't start until it emerges.

Getting a vaccine against a pandemic virus we know about may not be as easy as one might think. Vaccine manufacturing hasn't changed much since the 1976 swine flu panic, or, for that matter, since the 1940s. We still reproduce vaccine by growing it in eggs, a slow and costly process in the best of times. Once the pandemic virus makes it to the laboratory, it will take at least four months to create the vaccine, and six months is a more likely timeframe.

Adding to the problem is the fact that drug companies have no interest in manufacturing vaccines. The costs are high, the profits low, and the danger from lawsuits always present. In 2007 the U.S. licensed only three companies to do so. Three companies—none of them among the giant pharmaceutical corporations—simply can't produce the sheer volume of vaccine that'll be needed during a pandemic.

As the situation stands, there wouldn't be enough to go around, not in the U.S. and Europe, and not in poor countries. Yet getting the vaccine to people fast is vital because the body's immune system needs at least two weeks *after* a vaccination to generate antibodies. The Department of Health and Human Services plans to prioritize who gets vaccine, starting with health-care workers, then the elderly and those with chronic illness and compromised immune systems.

Of course, we have no idea where the next pandemic virus will come from. The fact is, many kinds of influenza circulate in the world. Within that are many kinds of avian influenza. Other subtypes of avian flu have infected human beings on rare occasions in the past. If one of them can improve its chances to survive by infecting us, it may mutate to do so and pull ahead of H5N1 on the list of threats. It's also possible one of the human influenza strains, like the H3N2s and H1N1s that cause illness today, could through antigenic drift or shift turn into a deadly virus.

The most significant influenza event since the 1997 avian flu outbreak came in March 2009. By April 23, the Centers for Disease Control confirmed seven cases of H1N1 influenza—trumpeted far and wide as "swine flu"—in the U.S. Laboratory tests indicated it was the same virus that had caused a spate of illness a month earlier in and near Mexico City.

Over the next week, cases appeared in multiple countries. The World Health Organization raised the warning level on its six-tiered pandemic alert system, first to Level Four and two days later to Five—the latter a warning of an imminent pandemic. Mexico City, one of the world's largest and most crowded urban environments, shut down. Schools were closed and three *futbol* (soccer) games were played in front of empty stadiums to limit the possible spread of disease.

Even as the city eased restrictions on May 5, twenty-one countries reported cases of H1N1. The figure rose to thirty-three countries on May 13, with 5,728 total cases. Of the fifty-three known deaths, forty-eight had occurred in Mexico, three in the U.S., and one each in Canada and Costa Rica. Attention, meanwhile, shifted to the Southern Hemisphere. There, the winter flu season was about to begin. Health officials prepared to track the virus's spread—and waited to see if it mutated into a more harmful form.

People around the world watch. And wait. The virus is always changing, the paths it takes complex and hard to follow, hard to even find much of the time. Influenza, with us for so long, is not going away.

Sources

CHAPTER ONE: Ever-Changing Virus

p. 19, "the vast majority . . ." Mike Davis, *The Monster at Our Door* (New York: New Press, 2005), 17.

CHAPTER TWO: Early History

p. 26, "he attacked the mules . . ." Homer, *The Illiad*, trans. E. V. Rieu, rev. ed. Peter Jones and D. C. H. Rieu (New York: Penguin, 2003), 3.

p. 27, "with difficulty . . ." George Rosen, *A History of Public Health* (Baltimore, MD: Johns Hopkins University Press, 1993), 21.

CHAPTER THREE: "Spanish Flu"

p. 37-38, "How many lives . . ." John M. Barry, *The Great Influenza* (New York: Penguin, 2005), 148.

p. 45, "the most vicious type . . ." Ibid., 187.

p. 45, "There was a man . . ." Rachel Wedeking, "A winding sheet and a wooden box" (interview with Josie Mabel Brown), *Navy Medicine* 77, no. 3 (May-June 1986): 18-19, Navy Department Library online at http://www.history.navy.mil/library/online/influenza%20wind.htm.

p. 47, "Pools of blood . . ." Alfred W. Crosby, *America's Forgotten Pandemic: The Influenza of 1918* (Cambridge: Cambridge University Press, 1989), 132.

CHAPTER FOUR: The Pandemic

p. 50-51, "[T]he 1918 virus . . ." Anne Underwood, "Resurrecting a killer flu," *Newsweek*, October 7, 2005, http://www.msnbc.msn.com/id/9623695/site/newsweek/.

p. 51, "There are very few . . ." Maryn McKenna, "Analysis of 1918 pandemic cites enduring mysteries," Center for Infectious Disease, Research, and Policy, March 6, 2007, http://www.cidrap.umn.edu/cidrap/content/influenza/panflu/news/mar0607fauci1918.html.

p. 56, "This will do much . . ." Crosby, *America's Forgotten Pandemic,* 74.

p. 58, "In essence . . ." National Institutes of Health press release, "Bacterial pneumonia caused most deaths in 1918 influenza pandemic," August 19, 2008, http://www.nih.gov/news/health/aug2008/niaid-19.htm.

p. 59, "Can send you . . . " Ibid., 51.

p. 61, "Some were delirious . . ." Wedeking, *Navy Medicine*, 18-19.

p. 62, "many died without . . ." Isaac Starr, "Influenza in 1918: Recollections of the epidemic in Philadelphia," *Annals of Internal Medicine* 145, no. 2 (July 18, 2006), http://www.annals.org/cgi/content/full/0000605 -200607180-00132v1.

p. 63, "When we left . . ." A. A. Hoehling, *The Great Epidemic* (Boston: Little, Brown, 1961), 163.

p. 66, "should not worry . . ." *New York Times,* "The Influenza," October 3, 1918.

p. 69, "It does not seem . . ." *New York Times,* "Tells of vaccine to stop influenza," October 2, 1918.

p. 69, "Our home at the time . . ." Richard Krause, "Swine Flu episode and the fog of epidemics," *Emerging Infectious Diseases* 12, no. 1 (January 2006): 40.

p. 75, "At the crest . . ." Associated Press, "Tahiti builds pyres of influenza dead," *New York Times*, December 25, 1918.

CHAPTER FIVE: Sneezing Ferrets and Swine Flu

p. 85, "I believe I have . . ." Gina Kolata, *Flu: The Story of the Great Influenza Pandemic of 1918 and the Search for the Virus That Caused It* (New York: Simon and Schuster, 1999), 68.

p. 86, "We have the technology . . ." Lauric Garrett, *The Coming Plague: Newly Emerging Diseases in a World Out of Balance* (New York: Penguin Books, 1994), 164.

p. 88, "[T]he possibility . . ." Ibid., 166.

p. 88, "Better a vaccine . . ." Kolata, *Flu*, 139.

p. 88, "By the time . . ." Philip M. Boffey, "Soft Evidence and hard sell," *New York Times Magazine*, September 5, 1976.

p. 90, "none of the vaccines . . ." Boffey, "Swine flu vaccination campaign: the scientific controversy mounts," *Science* 193, no. 4253 (August 13, 1976): 561.

CHAPTER SIX: H5N1

p. 102, "The important question . . ." Edward A. Gargan, "As avian flu spreads, China is seen as its epicenter," *New York Times*, December 21, 1997.

p. 107, "It suggests the virus . . ." Bernice Wuethrich, "An avian flu jumps to people," *Science* 299 (March 7, 2003): 1504.

p. 111, "The evidence is now overwhelming . . ." Debora MacKenzie, "Genes of deadly bird flu reveal Chinese origin," *New Scientist*, February 6, 2006, http://www.newscientist.com/article.ns?id=dn8686.

p. 120, "I sat on a pail . . ." Kolata, *Flu*, 262-63.

p. 123, "the most effective bioweapons . . ." "Special report: the 1918 flu virus is resurrected," *Nature* 437 (October 6, 2005): 794.

p. 123, "For the first time . . ." Underwood, "Resurrecting a killer flu."

CHAPTER SEVEN: Surveillance and Preparation

p. 132, "Under a moderate . . ." McKenna, "Analysis of 1918 pandemic."

p. 133, "The best defense . . ." Margaret Chan, address to World Health Day on international health security, World Health Organization document, April 2, 2007, http://www.who.int/dg/speeches/2007/020407_whd2007/en/index.html.

p. 136, "Pay attention to us . . ." Agus Maryono, "Chicken traders oppose mass culls to fight bird flu," *Jakarta Post*, January 29, 2007, http://www.thejakartapost.com/yesterdaydetail.asp?fileid=20070129.A05.

p. 143, "It's quite shocking . . ." Donald G. McNeil, Jr., "Major flu strain found resistant to leading drug, puzzling scientists," *New York Times,* January 9, 2009, http://www.nytimes.com/2009/01/09/health/09flu.html?partner=rss&emc=rss.

p. 143, "We could lose . . ." Kyung M. Song, *Seattle Times,* January 15, 2009, http://seattletimes.nwsource.com/html/health/2008630221_flu15m.html.

p. 145, "For years they have . . ." Elisabeth Rosenthal, "On the front: A pandemic is worrisome but 'unlikely,'" *New York Times*, March 28, 2006, http://www.nytimes.com/2006/03/28/health/28skep.html?ex=1301202000&en=c2e7fe90928b6dea&ei=5088.

Bibliography

BOOKS

Allen, Arthur. *Vaccine: The Controversial Story of Medicine's Greatest Lifesaver.* New York: W. W. Norton, 2007.

Barry, John M. *The Great Influenza.* New York: Penguin, 2005.

Beveridge, W. I. B. *Influenza: The Last Great Plague.* New York: Prodist, 1977.

Burnet, Macfarlane, and David O. White. *Natural History of Infectious Disease.* Cambridge: Cambridge University Press, 1972.

Byerly, Carol R. *Fever of War: The Influenza Epidemic in the U.S. Army.* New York: New York University Press, 2005.

Crosby, Alfred W. *America's Forgotten Pandemic: The Influenza of 1918.* Cambridge: Cambridge University Press, 1989.

Dallas, Gregor *1918: War and Peace.* Woodstock, NY: Overlook Press, 2001.

Davies, Pete. *The Devil's Flu.* New York: Henry Holt & Co., 1999.

Davis, Mike. *The Monster at Our Door.* New York: New Press, 2005.

Drexler, Madeline. *Secret Agents: The Menace of Emerging Infections.* Washington, D.C.: Joseph Henry Press, 2002.

Duncan, David Ewing. *Hernando de Soto: A Savage Quest in the Americas.* New York: Crown, 1995.

Farwell, Byron. *Over There: The United States in the Great War, 1917-18.* New York: W. W. Norton, 1999.

Garrett, Laurie. *The Coming Plague: Newly Emerging Diseases in a World Out of Balance.* New York: Penguin Books, 1994.

Givner, Joan. *Katherine Anne Porter: A Life.* New York: Simon and Schuster, 1982.

Greenfield, Karl Taro. *China Syndrome: The True Story of the 21st Century's First Great Epidemic.* New York: HarperCollins, 2006.

Greger, Michael. *Bird Flu: A Virus of Our Own Hatching.* New York: Lantern Books, 2006.

Hoehling, A. A. *The Great Epidemic.* Boston: Little, Brown, 1961.

Homer. *The Illiad.* Translated by E. V. Rieu. Edited by Peter Jones and D. C. H. Rieu. New York: Penguin, 2003.

Hudson, Charles. *The Southeastern Indians.* Knoxville, TN: University of Tennessee Press, 1976.

Karlen, Arno. *Man and Microbes.* New York: G. P. Putnam's Sons, 1995.

Keegan, John. *The First World War.* New York: Knopf, 1999.

Kolata, Gina. *Flu: The Story of the Great Influenza Pandemic of 1918 and the Search for the Virus that Caused It.* New York: Simon and Schuster, 1999.

Mann, Charles. *1491: New Revelations of the Americas Before Columbus.* New York: Knopf, 2005.

McNeill, William H. *Plagues and Peoples.* Garden City, NY: Anchor Press/Doubleday, 1976.

Persico, Joseph E. *11th Month, 11th Day, 11th Hour.* New York: Random House, 2004.

Porter, Katherine Anne. *Pale Horse, Pale Rider: Three Short Stories.* New York: Harcourt, Brace, Jovanovich, 1967.

Porter, Roy. *The Greatest Benefit to Mankind.* New York: W. W. Norton, 1997.

Rosen, George. *A History of Public Health.* Baltimore, MD: Johns Hopkins University Press, 1993.

Unrue, Darlene Harbour. *Katherine Anne Porter: Portrait of an Artist*. Jackson, Miss.: University Press of Mississippi, 2005.

Webster, Robert, and Scott Krauss, eds. *WHO Manual on Animal Diagnosis and Surveillance*. Geneva, Switzerland: World Health Organization, 2002.

Zelicoff, Alan P., and Michael Bellomo. *Microbe: Are We Ready for the Next Plague?* New York: Amacom, 2005.

PERIODICALS

Belshe, Robert B. "The origins of pandemic influenza—lessons from the 1918 virus." *New England Journal of Medicine* 353, no. 21 (November 24, 2005): 2209-2211.

Boffey, Philip M. "Guillan-Barré: Rare disease paralyzes swine flu campaign." *Science* 195, no. 4274 (January 14, 1977): 155-159.

———. "Soft evidence and hard sell." *New York Times Magazine*, September 5, 1976.

———. "Swine flu vaccination campaign: the scientific controversy mounts." *Science* 193, no. 4253 (August 13, 1976): 559-563.

Bradsher, Keith, and Lawrence K. Altman. "A war and a mystery: Confronting avian flu." *New York Times*, October 12, 2004.

Economist. "Coming home to roost?" January 27, 2007.

Enserink, Martin. "Oseltamivir becomes plentiful—but still not cheap." *Science* 312 (April 21, 2006): 382-383.

Fellows, Lawrence. "Hartford's elderly take their flu shots in stride." *New York Times*, October 15, 1976.

Ferris, P. "Flu: Sue nuisance, possible disaster." *New York Times Magazine*, January 11, 1976.

Gargan, Edward A. "As avian flu spreads, China is seen as its epicenter." *New York Times*, December 21, 1997.

Gibbs, W. Wayt, and Christine Soares. "Preparing for a pandemic." *Scientific American* 293, no. 5 (November 2005): 45-52, 54.

Kaiser, Jocelyn. "A one-size-fits-all flu vaccine?" *Science* 312 (April 21, 2006): 380-382.

Kobasa, Darwyn, Steven M. Jones, Kyoko Shinya, et al. "Aberrant innate immune response in lethal infection of macaques with the 1918 influenza virus." *Nature* 445 (January 18, 2007): 1319-323.

Krause, Richard. "The swine flu episode and the fog of epidemics." *Emerging Infectious Disease* 12, no. 1 (January 2006): 40-43.

Kuiken, Thijs, Edward C. Holmes, John McCauley, et al. "Host species barriers to influenza virus infections." *Science* 312 (April 21, 2006): 394-397.

Lederberg, Joshua. "H1N1 influenza as Lazarus." *Proceedings of the National Academy of Sciences* 98, no. 5 (February 27, 2001): 2115-2116.

Lu, Peter S. "Early diagnosis of avian influenza." *Science* 312 (April 26, 2006): 337.

Monto, Arnold S. "The threat of an avian influenza pandemic." *New England Journal of Medicine* 352, no. 4 (January 27, 2005): 323-325.

Morens, D. M., J. K. Taubenberger, and A. S. Fauci. "Predominant role of bacterial pneumonia as a cause of death in pandemic influenza: implications for pandemic influenza preparedness." *Journal of Infectious Disease* 198, no. 7 (October 1, 2008): 962-970.

Nature. "Special report: the 1918 flu virus is resurrected." *Nature*, 437 (October 6, 2005): 794-795.

New York Times. "Tahiti builds pyres of influenza dead." December 25, 1918.

————. "Tells of vaccine to stop influenza." October 2, 1918.

————. "4 p.m. close for most stores." October 5, 1918.

Osterholm, Michael T. "Unprepared for a pandemic."
Foreign Affairs 86, no. 2 (March-April, 2007): 47-57.

Public Health Reports. "Epidemic influenza and the
United States Public Health Service." *Public Health
Reports* 33, no. 43 (October 25, 1918): 378-380.

Sencer, David J., and J. Donald Miller. "Reflections on the
1976 swine flu vaccination program." *Emerging Infectious
Diseases* 12, no. 1 (January 2006): 29-33.

Smallman-Raynor, Matthew, and Andrew D. Cliff.
"Avian influenza A (H5N1) age distribution in humans."
Emerging Infectious Diseases 13, no. 3 (March
2007): 510-512.

Smith, Derek J. "Predictability and preparedness in influenza
control." *Science* 312 (April 21, 2006): 392-394.

Snacken, René, Alan P. Kendal, Lars R. Haaheim, et al.
"The next influenza pandemic: Lessons from Hong Kong,
1997." *Emerging Infectious Diseases* 5, no. 2 (March-April
1999): 195-201.

de Souza, Luciano Klebar, Marcus Panning, et al. "Spectrum
of viruses and atypical bacterial in intercontinental air
travelers with symptoms of acute respiratory infection."
Journal of Infectious Diseases 195 (January 18,
2007): 675-679.

Stevens, James, Ola Blixt, Terrence M. Tumpey, et al.,
"Structure and receptor specificity of the hemagglutinin
from an H5N1 influenza virus." *Science* 312 (April 21,
2006): 404-408.

Taubenberger, Jeffrey, and David M. Morens. "1918 influenza:
the mother of all pandemics." *Emerging Infectious
Diseases* 12, no. 1 (January 2006): 15-22.

Taubenberger, Morens, and Anthony S. Fauci. "The next influenza pandemic." *Journal of the American Medical Association* 297, no. 18 (May 9, 2007): 2025-2027.

Tumpey, Terence, Taronna R. Maines, Neal Van Hoeven, et al. "A two-amino acid change in the hemagglutinin of the 1918 influenza virus abolishes transmission." *Science* 315, no. 5812 (February. 2, 2007): 655-659.

Van Riel, Debby, Vincent J. Munster, Emmie de Wit, et al. "H5N1 virus attachment to lower respiratory tract." *Science* 312 (April 21, 2006): 399.

Webster, Malik Peiris, Honglin Chen, et al. "H5N1 outbreaks and enzootic influenza." *Emerging Infectious Diseases* 12, no. 1 (January 2006): 3-8.

Webster, Robert G., and Elena A. Govorkova. "H5N1 influenza—Continuing evolution and spread." *New England Journal of Medicine* 355, no. 21 (November 23, 2006): 2174-2177.

Winker, Kevin, Kevin G. McCracken, Daniel D. Gibson, et al., "Movements of birds and avian influenza from Asia into Alaska." *Emerging Infectious Diseases* 13, no. 4 (April 2007): 547-552.

World Health Organization Consultation on Human Influenza A/H5. "Avian influenza A (H5N1) infection in humans." *New England Journal of Medicine* 353, no. 13 (September 29, 2005): 1374-1385.

Wuethrich, Bernice. "An avian flu jumps to people." *Science* 299 (March 7, 2003): 1504.

———. "Chasing the fickle swine flu." *Science* 299 (March 7, 2003): 1502-1503, 1505.

ONLINE

Andrews, Mea. "Missoula readies for flu with look into past." *Missoulian*, January 21, 2006. http://www.missoulian.com/articles/2006/01/21/news/local/znews03.prt.

Armstrong, James F. "Philadelphia, nurses, and the Spanish Influenza pandemic of 1918." *Navy Medicine* 92, no. 2 (March-April 2001): 16-20. http://www.history.navy.mil/library/online/influenza%20phil%201918.htm.

Bakalar, Nicholas. "How (and how not) to battle flu: A tale of 23 cities." *New York Times*, April 17, 2007. http://www.nytimes.com/2007/04/17/health/17flu.html?ex=1180065600&en=302e807ff91ee820&ei=5070.

Barrett, Jennifer. "Why you should worry about avian flu." *Newsweek*, September 30, 2005. http://www.msnbc.msn.com/id/9547047/site/newsweek/.

Batty, David. "Experts slam government's flu outbreak plans." *Guardian*, May 11, 2007. http://society.guardian.co.uk/health/story/0,,2077735,00.html.

Beck, Lindsey. "China shares bird flu samples, denies new strain report." *Reuters AlertNet*, November 10, 2006. http://www.alertnet.org/thenews/newsdesk/PEK2663.htm.

Blankinship, Donna Gordon. "Washington uses flu pandemic money to prepare for any disaster." Associated Press, December 17, 2006. http://seattlepi.nwsource.com/local/6420/AP_WA_Pandemic_Readiness_Wash.html.

Borenstein, Seth. "1918 flu killed by turning the body against itself." Associated Press, January 17, 2007. http://www.usatoday.com/tech/science/discoveries/flu-research.htm?POE=NEWISVA.

Brown, David. "A shot in the dark: swine flu's vaccine lessons." *Washington Post*, May 27, 2002. http://www.washingtonpost.com/ac2/wp-dyn/A14517-2002.

————. "Masks' flu protection assessed." *Washington Post*, April 28, 2006. http://www.sfgate.com/cgi-bin/article. cgi?file=/c/a/2006/04/28/MNGPKIGRJH1.DTL.

————. "World not set to deal with flu." *Washington Post*, July 31, 2005. http://www.washingtonpost.com/wp-dyn/ content/article/2005/07/30/AR2005073001429.html.

Callaway, Ewen. "Bacteria were the real killers in 1918 flu pandemic." *New Scientist,* August 4, 2008. http://www. newscientist.com/article/dn14458-bacteria-were-the-real-killers-in-1918-flu-pandemic.html.

Center for Infections Disease, Research, and Policy. "Avian Influenza (Bird Flu): Implications for Human Disease." http://www.cidrap.umn.edu/cidrap/content/influenza/ avianflu/biofacts/avflu_human.html.

Chan, Margaret. Address to World Health Day on international health security, World Health Organization document, April 2, 2007. http://www.who.int/dg/speeches/2007/ 020407_whd2007/en/index.html.

Chong, Winnie. "Bird flu sparks renewed calls on poultry sales." *Standard* (Hong Kong), March 22, 2007. http://www.thestandard.com.hk/news_detail.asp?we_ cat=4&art_id=40704&sid=12773076&con_type=1.

Colizza, Victoria, Alain Barrat, Marc Barthelemy, et al. "Modeling the worldwide spread of pandemic influenza: Baseline case and containment interventions." *PloS Medicine* 4, no. 1 (January 23, 2007). http://medicine.plosjournals.org/ archive/1549-1676/4/1/pdf/10.1371_journal.pmed.0040013-S.pdf.

Cortazal, Manuel. "Preparing for pandemic." *Boston Globe*, March 17, 2006. http://www.boston.com/news/globe/ editorial_opinion/oped/articles/2006/03/17/preparing_for_ pandemic/.

Eban, Katherine. "Biosense or biononsense?" *Scientist* 21, no. 4 (April 2007). http://www.the-scientist.com/article/ daily/52963/.

Food and Agricultural Organization of the United Nations. "Should wild birds now be considered a permanent reservoir of the virus?" *FAO Avian Influenza Disease Emergency*, no. 40, June 19, 2006. http://www.fao.org/docs/eims/upload/209858/AVIbull040.pdf.

Fox, Maggie. "Bird flu hard to detect until too late—studies." *Reuters AlertNet*, November 22, 2006. http://www.alertnet.org/thenews/newsdesk/N22213059.htm.

————. "Bird imports may spread bird flu in Americas—study." *Reuters AlertNet*, December 4, 2006. http://www.alertnet.org/thenews/newsdesk/N04489802.htm.

————. "Flu viruses survive frozen in lakes, study finds." *Reuters AlertNet*, November 28, 2006. http://www.alertnet.org/thenews/newsdesk/N28291567.htm.

————. "Tamiflu maker lowers production, says slow demand." *Reuters AlertNet*, April 26, 2007. http://www.alertnet.org/thenews/newsdesk/L26435875.htm.

Garrett, Laurie. "The next pandemic?" *Foreign Affairs*, July-August 2005. http://www.foreignaffairs.org/20050701faessay84401/laurie-garrett/the-next-pandemic.html.

Gernhart, Gary. "A Forgotten Enemy: PHS's Fight Against the 1918 Influenza Pandemic." *Public Health Reports* (November-December 1999): 559-561. Navy Department Library online. http://www.history.navy.mil/library/online/influenza_forgot.htm.

Griffith, Dorsey, and Edie Lau. "State readies pandemic response." *Sacramento Bee*, January 19, 2006. http://www.sacbee.com/content/news/ongoing/flu/v-print/story/14090823p-14920808c.html.

Handwerk, Brian. "Bird flu strain diversified, may be harder to conquer." National Geographic News, February 7, 2006. http://news.nationalgeographic.com/news/2006/02/0207_060207_bird_flu.html.

Hawley, David. "Could next outbreak rival 1918 flu?" *Minneapolis Pioneer Press*, November 26, 2006. http://www.twincities. com/mld/pioneerpress/news/local/16091793.htm.

Kawana, Akihiko, Go Naka, Yuji Fujikura, et al. "Spanish influenza in Japanese armed forces, 1918-1920." *Emerging Infectious Diseases*, April 2007. http://www.cdc.gov/eid/ content/13/4/590.htm.

Kirkey, Sharon. "Bird flu's deadly shadows of 1918." CanWest News Service, January 27, 2006. http://www. canada.com/nationalpost/news/bodyandhealth/story. html?id=a5c966cb-74c2-45ba-b981-6ce0477fa5fa.

Kolata, Gina. "The 1918 flu killed millions. Does it hold clues for today?" *New York Times*, March 28, 2006. http://topics. nytimes.com/2006/03/28/science/28flu.html.

Larson, Erik. "The flu hunters." *Time*, February 23, 1998. http:// www.time.com/time/magazine/article/0,9171,987857,00. html.

Lauerman, John. "Novartis, Sanofi seek universal influenza vaccine." *Bloomberg*, December 11, 2006. http://www. bloomberg.com/apps/news?pid=20670001&rcfcr=europe &sid=avDqqU1J2AZw.

Levy, Adrian, and Cathy Scott-Clark. "Flu on the wing." *Guardian*, October 15, 2005. http://www.guardian.co.uk/ birdflu/story/0,14207,1591358,00.html.

MacKenzie, Debora. "Early human bird flu death uncovered in China." *New Scientist*, June 22, 2006. http://www. newscientist.com/article/dn9388-early-human-bird-flu-death-uncovered-in-china.html.

———. "Genes of deadly bird flu reveal Chinese origin." *New Scientist*, February 6, 2006. http://www.newscientist. com/article.ns?id=dn8686.

———. "Nigeria's strain of bird flu bode ill for Africa." *New Scientist*, July 5, 2006. http://www.newscientist. com/article.ns?id=mg19125594.200.

————. "WHO lab confirms Iraqi bird flu death."
New Scientist, February 1, 2006. http://www.newscientist.
com/article.ns?id=dn8664.

Manning, Anita. "The great flu pandemic: Despite dire
warnings, public interest has waned." *USA Today*,
February 1, 2007. http://www.usatoday.com/news/health/
2007-01-31-great-flu-pandemic_x.htm.

Marsa, Linda. "Fighting the bird flu, fast," *Los Angeles Times,*
January 29, 2007. http://www.latimes.com/features/health/
la-he-lab29jan29,1,3832186.story?coll=la-headlines-health.

Maryono, Agus. "Chicken traders oppose mass culls to fight
bird flu." *Jakarta Post*, January 29, 2007. http://www.the
jakartapost.com/yesterdaydetail.asp?fileid=20070129.A05.

McAnally, W. F. "Influenza on a naval transport." *United
States Medical Bulletin* 13, no. 1: 168-170. Navy Department
Library, http://www.history.navy.mil/library/online/
influenza_transport.htm.

McKenna, Maryn. "Analysis of 1918 pandemic cites enduring
mysteries." Center for Infectious Disease, Research,
and Policy, March 6, 2007. http://www.cidrap.umn.
edu/cidrap/content/influenza/panflu/news/mar0607
fauci1918.html.

————. "Social distancing helped some cities endure 1918
pandemic." Center for Infectious Disease, Research,
and Policy, April 3, 2007. http://www.cidrap.umn.edu/cidrap/
content/influenza/panflu/news/apr0307mitigate.html.

————. "Review finds little evidence of airborne spread of
flu." Center for Infectious Disease, Research, and Policy,
March 13, 2007. http://www.cidrap.umn.edu/cidrap/
content/influenza/general/news/mar1307transmit.html.

McNeil, Donald Jr. "Bird flu's risks far from over, experts
warn." *International Herald-Tribune*, February 14, 2007.
http://www.iht.com/articles/2007/02/14/news/flu.php.

————. "Closing and cancellations top advice on flu outbreak." *New York Times*, February 2, 2007. http://www.nytimes.com/2007/02/02/health/02flu.html?ex=1180065600&en=f8fcb972128bc6f3&ei=5070.

————. "Major flu strain found resistant to leading drug, puzzling scientists." *New York Times,* January 9, 2009. http://www.nytimes.com/2009/01/09/health/09flu.html?partner=rss&emc=rss.

————. "New strain of bird flu found in Egypt is resistant to antiviral drug." *New York Times*, January 18, 2007. http://select.nytimes.com/gst/abstract.html?res=F00C17FB3A540C7B8DDDA80894DF404482.

————. "Scientists hope vigilance stymies avian flu mutations." *New York Times*, March 27, 2007. http://www.nytimes.com/2007/03/27/health/27flu.html?ex=1180065600&en=81339a57d69ec825&ei=5070.

National Institutes of Health. "Bacterial pneumonia caused most deaths in 1918 influenza pandemic." Press release, August 19, 2008. http://www.nih.gov/news/health/aug2008/niaid-19.htm.

————. "New study has important implications for influenza surveillance, vaccine formulation." Press release, October 25, 2006. http://www.nih.gov/news/pr/oct2006/nlm-25.htm.

————. "Rapid response was crucial to containing the 1918 flu pandemic." Press release, April 2, 2007. http://www3.niaid.nih.gov/news/newsreleases/2007/fluresponse.htm.

National Museum of Health and Medicine. "Images from the 1918 influenza epidemic." http://nmhm.washingtondc.museum/collections/archives/agalleries/1918flu/1918flu.html.

Nebehay, Stephanie. "China shares bird flu samples in 'breakthrough'—WHO." *Reuters AlertNet*, September 28, 2006. http://www.alertnet.org/thenews/newsdesk/L28693486.

Neergaard, Lauran. "Bird flu gene analysis finds new clue." Associated Press, January 26, 2006. http://www.sfgate. com/cgi-bin/article.cgi?f=/n/a/2006/01/26/national/ a110144S09.DTL.

Nesbitt, Jim. "When killer flu struck." *News and Observer*, November 26, 2006. http://www.newsobserver.com/ 105/story/514837.html.

Oo, Aung Lwin. "The invisible enemy." *Irrawaddy* 15, no. 5 (May 2007). http://www.irrawaddymedia.com/article. php?art_id=7107.

Orent, Wendy. "Worrying about killer flu." *Discovery*, February 25, 2005. http://discovermagazine.com/2005/ feb/worrying-about-killer-flu.

Paseka, Nicole. "Remembering a killer." *Sioux City Journal*, March 18, 2007. http://www.siouxcityjournal.com/articles/ 2007/03/18/news/top/8851550f7e83485d862572a200136b39.txt.

Pearson, Helen. "Controlling immune response may cut bird flu death rate." *Nature Medicine*, September 8, 2006. http:// www.nature.com/news/2006/060904/full/nm1493.html.

Perrin, Andrew. "Playing chicken." *Time*, January 26, 2004. http://www.time.com/time/magazine/article/0,9171, 582473,00.html.

Phouthonesy, Ekaphone. "Bird flu control needs public cooperation." *Vientiane Times*, March 7, 2007. http://www. vientianetimes.org.la/FreeContent/FreeContent_bird.htm.

Pincock, Stephen. "And if bird flu hits Africa . . ." *Scientist*, January 20, 2006. http://www.the-scientist.com/news/ display/22989/.

Pollack, Andrew. "Lessons from a plague that wasn't." *New York Times*, October 23, 2005. http://www. nytimes.com/2005/10/23/weekinreview/23pollack. html?ex=1180065600&en=2c7ee32be02f5f63&ei=5070.

Reynolds, Gretchen. "The flu hunters." *New York Times Magazine*, November 7, 2004. http://www.nytimes.com/2004/11/07/magazine/07FLU.html?ex=1180152000&en=3a5b12301ba136ce&ei=5070.

Roos, Robert. "NIH: 2,000 flu viruses sequenced, data published." Center for Infectious Disease, Research, and Policy, February 22, 2007. http://www.cidrap.umn.edu/cidrap/content/influenza/general/news/feb2207genome.html.

———. "Study: Bacterial pneumonia was main killer in 1918 flu pandemic." August 22, 2008. http://www.cidrap.umn.edu/cidrap/content/influenza/panflu/news/aug2208pneumo.html.

Rosenthal, Elisabeth. "Bird flu reports multiply in Turkey, faster than expected." *New York Times*, January 9, 2006. http://www.nytimes.com/2006/01/09/international/europe/09flu.html?ex=1180065600&en=20a9924eac9b4230&ei=5070.

———. "On the front: A pandemic is worrisome but 'unlikely'." *New York Times*, March 28, 2006. http://www.nytimes.com/2006/03/28/health/28skep.html?ex=1301202000&en=c2e7fe90928b6dea&ei=5088.

Rosenwald, Michael. "The flu hunter." *Smithsonian*, January 2006. http://www.smithsonianmag.com/issues/2006/january/flu.php.

Roylance, Frank D. "Bird flu trackers focus on Alaska." *Hartford Courant*, March 6, 2006. http://www.courant.com/news/nationworld/hc-alaska0306.artmar06,0,1114372.story?coll=hc=headlines-nationworld.

Schnirring, Lisa. "Egypt finds more H5N1 in poultry." Center for Infectious Disease, Research, and Policy. January 22, 2009. http://www.cidrap.umn.edu/cidrap/content/influenza/avianflu/news/jan2209avian-br.html.

————. "H5N1 hits Nepal for the first time, strikes another Indian state." Center for Infectious Disease, Research, and Policy. January 22, 2009. http://www.cidrap.umn.edu/cidrap/content/influenza/avianflu/news/jan2009avian.html.

————. "Indonesia quits offering prompt notice of H5N1 cases." Center for Infectious Disease, Research, and Policy, June 5, 2008. http://www.cidrap.umn.edu/cidrap/content/influenza/avianflu/news/jun0508indonesia-br.html.

Schnirring, Lisa, and Robert Roos. "FDA approves first H5N1 vaccine." Center for Infectious Disease, Research, and Policy, April 17, 2007. http://www.cidrap.umn.edu/cidrap/content/influenza/avianflu/news/apr1707vaccine.html.

Sharma, Gopal. "Nepal reports first H5N1 bird flu outbreak." *Reuters,* January 16, 2009. http://www.alertnet.org/thenews/newsdesk/DEL133818.htm.

Sheridan, Barrett. "The threat from China's pigs." *Newsweek*, May 10, 2006. http://www.msnbc.msn.com/id/18597469/site/newsweek/.

Smith, Nicole, Joseph S. Bresee, David K. Shay, et al. "Prevention and Control of Influenza: Recommendations of the Advisory Committee on Influenza Practices." *Morbidity and Mortality Weekly Report*, July 28, 2006. http://www.cdc.gov/mmwr/preview/mmwrhtml/rr5510a1.htm.

Song, Kyung M. "One major flu strain resistant to Tamiflu treatment." *Seattle Times,* January 15, 2009. http://seattletimes.nwsource.com/html/health/2008630221_flu15m.html.

Springer, Patrick. "101-year-old recalls 1918 flu epidemic." Associated Press, April 27, 2007. http://customwire.ap.org/dynamic/stories/N/ND_1918_FLU_NDOL-?SITE=WIWAT&SECTION=US&TEMPLATE=DEFAULT&CTIME=2007-04-27-15-48-43.

Starr, Isaac. "Influenza in 1918: Recollections of the epidemic in Philadelphia." *Annals of Internal Medicine* 145, no. 2 (July 18, 2006). http://www.annals.org/cgi/content/full/0000605-200607180-00132v1.

Taubenberger, Jeffrey K., and Jared Lipworth. Online chat, *Washington Post*, November 22, 2005. http://www.washingtonpost.com/wp-dyn/content/discussion/2005/11/21/DI2005112100469.html.

Taubenberger, Jeffery K., and Kurt Tondorf. Online chat, *Washington Post*, March 4, 2004. http://www.washingtonpost.com/ac2/wp-dyn/A23473-2004Mar2?language=printer.

Tre, Tuoi, trans. by Hoang Bao. "Chinese fowl still imported during bird flu insurgence." *Thanh Nien News*, January 3, 2007. http://www.thanhniennews.com/print.php?catid=10&newsid=23846.

Underwood, Anne. "Resurrecting a killer flu." *Newsweek* (online), October 7, 2005. http://www.msnbc.msn.com/id/9623695/site/newsweek/.

United Nations Office for the Coordination of Humanitarian Affairs. "Nigeria: The poor the weakest link as bird flu bites." Integrated Regional Information Networks, February 27, 2007. http://www.irinnews.org/Report.aspx?ReportId=70435.

U.S. Department of Health and Human Services: Pandemic Influenza Plan. http://www.hhs.gov/pandemicflu/plan/.
———. Pandemic planning update. http://www.pandemicflu.gov/plan/pdf/panflu20060313.pdf.

U.S. Food and Drug Administration. "FDA approves first U.S. vaccine for humans against avian influenza virus H5N1." Press release, April 17, 2007. http://www.fda.gov/bbs/topics/NEWS/2007/NEW01611.html.

U.S. Navy Department Library. "The influenza epidemic
of 1918." Photo gallery, undated. http://www.history.navy.
mil/photos/events/ev-1910s/ev-1918/influenz.htm.

Walsh, Bryan. "Indonesia's bird flu showdown." *Time*,
May 10, 2007. http://www.time.com/time/health/article/
0,8599,1619229,00.html.

Wedeking, Rachel. "A winding sheet and a wooden box."
Interview with Josie Mabel Brown, *Navy Medicine* 77,
no. 3 (May-June 1986): 18-19. Navy Department Library
online, http://www.history.navy.mil/library/online/
influenza%20wind.htm.

World Health Organization. "Cumulative number of confirmed
human cases of avian influenza A/(H5N1) reported to WHO."
May 16, 2007. http://www.who.int/csr/disease/avian_
influenza/country/cases_table_2007_05_16/en/.

————. Global Influenza Surveillance Network. http://www.
who.int/csr/disease/influenza/surveillance/en/.

————. "Monitoring of neuraminidase inhibitor resistance
among clinical influenza isolates in Japan during
2003-2006 influenza seasons." *Weekly Epidemiological
Record* 82, no. 17 (April 27, 2007): 149-150. http://www.
who.int/wer/2007/wer8217/en/print.html.

Web sites

http://www.cdc.gov/flu/avian/
The Center for Disease Control's page about Avian flu. Features key facts about the disease, as well as information for those traveling abroad who might be exposed to the disease, and up-to-date information about treatments.

http://www.cidrap.umn.edu/cidrap/content/influenza/ avianflu/
The University of Minnesota's Center for Infectious Disease Research and Policy's page on avian flu. Features current news on the disease, its treatments, and pages devoted to the topics of biosecurity, food safety, and the threat of bioterrorism.

http://www.pandemicflu.gov/
Web site devoted to gathering the U.S. Government's information about the pandemic and avian flu. Features information about government health policies, global outbreaks, the economic impact of the diseases, and links for fighting the disease in the community.

http://ec.europa.eu/food/animal/diseases/controlmeasures/ avian/index_en.htm
The European Union's page about avian flu, and its effects throughout Europe, as well information about European efforts to fight the infection.

http://www.who.int/csr/disease/influenza/en/
The World Health Organization's page about the flu, featuring recommendations for vaccines, FAQs, and information about pandemic preparedness.

http://www.who.int/csr/disease/avian_influenza/ai_time line/en/index.html
The World Health Organization's detailed timeline of avian influenza's appearance and infections throughout the world.

Glossary

antigenic drift
Antigenic drift is the process of ongoing mutation in an influenza virus's genetic structure that gradually alters its genetic code and shape.

antigenic shift
An antigenic shift takes place when a sudden change in an influenza virus's genetic structure allows influenza from one species (for example, birds) to leap to another (for example, pigs or humans.)

endemic
Endemic means constantly present in an area or country.

epidemic
An epidemic is a sharp increase in the number of cases of a disease, whether in an area where the disease exists or in an area where it's unknown.

hemagglutinin
One of the two major proteins on the surface of an influenza virus. Hemagglutinin hooks onto and unlocks an animal cell, allowing the virus to get inside. Hemagglutinin is abbreviated to HA or H.

neuraminidase (NA or N)
One of the two main proteins on the surface of an influenza virus. Neuraminidase neutralizes chemicals on the surface of a human cell, allowing copies of influenza virus to escape and spread. Neuraminidase is abbreviated to NA or N.

pathogen
A disease-causing virus, bacteria, parasite, or other organism.

pandemic
A series of epidemics taking place over a large area of the world.

reassortment
The process influenza viruses use to trade genes and create new hybrid viruses.

selection pressure
Selection pressure takes place when an outside factor (or group of factors) encourages a virus or living organism to adapt or mutate as a way to survive.

subtype
Subtypes are families of influenza viruses classified according to their hemagglutinin and neuraminidase proteins. The thousands of viruses within a subtype can have considerable differences in genetic structure.

Index